ACCESS YOUR ONLINE RESOURCES

Navigating Telehealth for Speech and Language Therapists is accompanied by a number of printable online materials, designed to ensure this resource best supports your professional needs

Activate your online resources:
Go to www.routledge.com/cw/speechmark and click on the cover of this book
Click the 'Sign in or Request Access' button and follow the instructions in order to access the resources

I0032192

NAVIGATING TELEHEALTH FOR SPEECH AND LANGUAGE THERAPISTS

There is so much to consider in any clinical consultation: identifying the individual is the one you expected, who is with the individual, which therapy intervention, resources, signposting, referrals, being cued in to responses for contextual information, evaluation and outcomes, planning next steps … and this is all before you throw 'virtual' in the mix!

This clinical companion presents 50 transferable, adaptable, practical and accessible chapters for speech and language therapists and others working via remote consultations.

Divided into four sections, the book covers:

- The remote practitioner.
- The remote rules.
- Creating a digital tool kit.
- A remotely possible future.

Aimed at students encountering their first remote consultations, newly qualified clinicians with limited practical experience of virtual clinics through to clinicians who are experienced in their own specialities but now need to transfer those skills to remote ways of delivery, this concise text will provide confidence and guidance for the reader. It will also prove useful to clinicians beyond speech and language as many of the skills and practical advice and guidance are applicable in specialities across a range of settings, both public and private, healthcare and education.

Rebekah Davies is a speech and language therapist with over 14 years of clinical experience. She is the co-author of the RCSLT Telehealth Guidance, a Topol Digital Health Fellow and a member of the Faculty of Clinical Informatics and NHS Digital Academy.

Navigating Telehealth for Speech and Language Therapists

Navigating the field of speech and language therapy can seem overwhelming to students and newly qualified therapists. This series is designed to provide concise, entry level summaries of key areas in speech and language therapy, providing a basic insight into a specific area of therapy. Comprising practical advice and guidance from an expert in the field, the books cover topics such as assessment, therapy, psychological approaches and onward referral. This is a useful tool for anyone new to speech and language therapy or building confidence in their field.

NAVIGATING ADULT STAMMERING
100 Points for Speech and Language Therapists
Trudy Stewart

NAVIGATING TELEHEALTH FOR SPEECH AND
LANGUAGE THERAPISTS
The Remotely Possible in 50 Key Points
Rebekah Davies

NAVIGATING TELEHEALTH FOR SPEECH AND LANGUAGE THERAPISTS

THE REMOTELY POSSIBLE IN 50 KEY POINTS

Rebekah Davies

Routledge
Taylor & Francis Group

LONDON AND NEW YORK

First published 2023
by Routledge
4 Park Square, Milton Park, Abingdon, Oxon, OX14 4RN

and by Routledge
605 Third Avenue, New York, NY 10158

Routledge is an imprint of the Taylor & Francis Group, an informa business

© 2023 Rebekah Davies

British Library Cataloguing-in-Publication Data
A catalogue record for this book is available from the British Library

Library of Congress Cataloging-in-Publication Data
A catalog record has been requested for this book

ISBN: 978-1-032-21719-2 (hbk)
ISBN: 978-1-032-21720-8 (pbk)
ISBN: 978-1-003-26972-4 (ebk)

DOI: 10.4324/9781003269724

Typeset in Aldus
by Deanta Global Publishing Services, Chennai, India

Access the companion website: www.routledge.com/cw/speechmark

This book is dedicated to my much-loved family and with special dedication to the man who knew something about everything: 'Prof'! He was my Grandad, my hero and my greatest champion, with whom I have a special bond that will remain unbroken by time and space. Love always, RV x

CONTENTS

Section 3
THE REMOTE TOOLS: CREATING A DIGITAL TOOLKIT

Section 4
A REMOTELY POSSIBLE FUTURE

GLOSSARY OF TERMS

AHPIO – Allied Health Professional Information Officer: an informatics role undertaken by an Allied Health Professional to support the AHP workforce with digital transformation and informatics workstreams across an organisation. Limited in instance, sometimes referred to as CAHPIO where the 'C' indicates Chief. Often a CNIO will undertake the responsibility for AHPs as well as nurses, an area in hot discussion amongst the informatics AHP workforce as it is felt only an AHP can represent other AHPs effectively.

API – Application Programming Interface: in simple terms it's a gateway to allow one system or piece of tech to 'talk' or pass information to another. These are *really* useful in healthcare where we need to share information securely and easily between two systems or more as data/information can be 'pushed' or sent between the two, provided the API or gateway is open and allows the information to exit or enter. This is one example of how electronic data is shared between systems.

Application (app): a piece of software downloaded from the app store on a mobile device for a range of purposes from video consultation platforms to therapy assessments or remote monitoring tools to use between therapy sessions.

Asynchronous: completing digital healthcare activities outside of the standard appointment, such as a remote monitoring questionnaire. The converse is synchronous.

CIO – Chief Information Officer: a CIO leads the digital agenda in addition to overseeing the hardware, software and data that helps other members of both the health informatics directorate and wider organisation in leading and researching new technologies, strategising how technology can provide business value and support clinical and governance leads address associated digital information and clinical risk mitigation.

CCIO – Chief Clinical Information Officer: support the CIO to deliver the clinical element of the digital transformation agenda by working with the clinical workforce, understanding the challenges faced by clinicians.

CNIO – Chief Nursing Information Officer: similar in remit to the CCIO but specific to the nursing workforce; however, in some organisations, the CNIO can also be responsible for AHPs, which has been the source of some discussion as this is felt to be unrepresentative of the professions due to the difference between the roles.

CXIO – Chief (insert title) Information Officer: as with CCIO or CNIO roles, the 'X' represents any other clinical or non-clinical role in the informatics field, so it can be CDIO, which could be Chief Digital or Chief Dental Information Officer, Chief Ethics and Data, Chief Privacy, Chief Technology, Chief Allied Health Professional and any number of others could be created to fit a particular clinical speciality if CCIO.

CHiME – College of Healthcare Information Management Executives: a US-based informatics company with UK affiliation and providing sought-after accreditation by CIOs working in healthcare to become accredited Certified Health CIOs (CHCIO) by undertaking an exam to prove their skills and competence in the area.

Clinical Informatics: a profession that utilises technology and data to support safer, more efficient and innovative healthcare reports for the DCB 129 and 160 standards to clinically assure new and existing technologies and mitigate risks that could impact patient safety.

Digital Practice: the act of practising using digital tools or means.

Digital Practitioner: an individual who uses digital tools to practise (such as virtual consultations).

DTAC – Digital Technology Assessment Criteria: an assurance framework for digital tools laid out in 2020 by NHSE/I Transformation Directorate (formerly NHSX) for all suppliers of health tech solutions.

DPO – Data Protection Officer: an individual that works within an organisation and leads on data and cyber security, largely but exclusively aligned to the protection of personal data.

FCI – Faculty of Clinical Informatics: a professional standards body for the accreditation of clinicians working within the clinical informatics arena. Membership is at three levels, associate, member and fellow with various bursaries available to encourage underrepresented groups, including BAME through the Shuri Network.

FedIP – Federation of Informatics Professionals: a professional standards body that is for all professionals working in health informatics seeking accreditation.

HEE – Health Education England: the national body which supports the digital readiness programme alongside NHS England and Improvement and also develops and delivers national training and guidance for the health and social care workforce.

Individuals: people, patients, pupils, students, patients, citizens, public, service users.

Information Governance (IG): the overall strategy for information at an organisation. Typically a small department, often with an information governance (IG) lead or manager alongside the DPO and Caldicott lead for the organisation to protect public information being shared with other members of the public. Information governance balances the risk that information presents with the value that information provides. Information governance helps with legal compliance, operational transparency, and reducing expenditures associated with legal discovery.

In-person: face-to-face appointment in a traditional clinic setting or home visit.

NHS Digital: a national arm's length body of the NHS responsible for the NHS mail, NHS App and many of the digital policies nationally that SLTs use.

NHS England and NHS Improvement: two directorates combined in 2019 to form one strategic directorate. This arm drives the main agenda for outpatient and primary care transformation nationally, with regional support divided across each geographical area and each region overseeing a series of integrated care systems (ICS).

NHSE/I Transformation Directorate (formerly known as NHSX): a national body made up of professionals from NHS England and Improvement and the Department of Health and Social Care. Their premise is to support healthcare systems with digital transformation by,

1. Negotiating national-level contracts, including funding for new projects.
2. Design the technical architecture to link up the whole system across health and care.
3. Set national policy to deliver the necessary change.

NHSE/I Transformation Directorate (formerly NHSX) sets the overall strategy for digital transformation and they commission a further national arm, NHS Digital, to deliver existing APIs to the NHS Spine and National Record Locator Service.

All three arms will be operating under the NHS England and Improvement banner to further streamline digital transformation, limit duplication of guidance and reduce silos of work happening nationally to make the national digital engine more efficient.

ORCHA: an organisation that reviews and assures health apps against the DTAC standards and offers support to healthcare organisations for libraries of apps specific to conditions.

PIFU – Patient-Initiated Follow Up: a method of caseload management to support patients receiving timely and efficient care and virtual/video consultations may be used as part of this pathway.

Platform: a piece of software to deliver a video call or may be hybrid and allow 'soft telephone' on screen via a dial pad. Many platforms are on the market, although a few are better-known and more readily approved in healthcare than others.

Remote Consultation: usually refers to video but can include consultations or episodes of care that utilise apps.

Remote Monitoring: the use of digital tools, including asynchronous telehealth tools, such as patient-facing apps where the patient logs in and records specific qualitative information (for example, in voice therapy it may be set around reaching a more feminine pitch using an app such as Christella). These may be a combination of exercises pre-set by a therapist and signposting to online videos and exercises. There may be a two-way ability allowing an individual to leave or send updates, videos and images for their clinician between therapy sessions which can be recorded for progress in their patient record. Wearable devices may also be included in remote monitoring to capture data.

Shuri Network: BAME community of women in health tech who welcome allies from across the health tech sector.

Synchronous: completing digital/virtual care activities such as video consultations in real time, converse is asynchronous.

Telecare/ Teleconsultation/ Telehealth/ Telemedicine/ Telepractice/ Teletherapy: A healthcare consultation conducted using non-face -to -face methods covers all 'tele'-prefixed consults. These may be either telephone,video or hybrid. The latter starts as a telephone call transfers to a video call or vice versa.

Virtual Consultations: umbrella terms for telephone and video consultations. Data can be related to either contact type and national guidance does not define the difference (2021).

Video Consultations: relates specifically to video consultations, although many organisations have struggled to report accurately on video.

WCAG – Web Content Accessibility Guidelines: developed through the W3C (World Wide Web Continuum) process in cooperation with individuals and organisations around the world, with a goal of providing a single shared standard for web content accessibility that meets the needs of individuals, organisations, and governments internationally.

The WCAG standards highlight that any information available on the web or more recently in mobile applications,

1. Provide text alternatives for non-text content.
2. Provide captions and other alternatives for multimedia.
3. Create content that can be presented in different ways, including by assistive technologies, without losing meaning.
4. Make it easier for users to see and hear content.

INTRODUCTION: THE REMOTEST POSSIBILITY

If you are looking for practical guidance following the end to end journey of a digital practitioner; steering and helping to navigate clinicians who are complete virtual virgins through uncharted screens and clicks, whilst providing content-rich tips and tricks for those already more confident in their use of virtual medium for therapy, then this is the book for you.

It's not a book or handbook to cite, it's a book to have in your sights and in your hand!

Writing this during a pandemic that has been ongoing, affecting my own life and the lives of those around me so deeply has been both a challenge and a privilege, highlighting that, even when things seem impossible, speech and language therapists (SLT) succeed to enable and empower even where there may be just the remotest possibility. I hope wherever you are in your journey you find something that helps you navigate your digital delivery with more confidence and competence than before.

DOI: 10.4324/9781003269724-1

THE REMOTE
PRACTITIONER

NEW TO DIGITAL PRACTICE: THE PRACTICALITIES

First of all, welcome! Please be reassured however new you are too digital practice, you are not the only one. For many, digital felt and still can feel like it is something that has been done to them, not something they have wholeheartedly agreed to. I was a little different as I had already begun my digital journey prior to the onslaught of Covid-19, but I quickly realised for many that this just wasn't the case. Overnight, 'virtual' was a word that appeared and suddenly the expectation was that our caseloads were suddenly online, as were the people to which the name belonged.

There were and are so many practicalities to get your head around, from whether your computer can even do a virtual appointment to wondering if all the person on the other side of the screen can see is the top of your head or your bottom jaw. Getting a chair to fit the bill was half the problem, and if that wasn't viable maybe a table with a couple of books under each leg to alter the height. I've tried it all! Most of it with limited success and a huge amount of frustration and that, for me, is where the premise of this book is built from, experience. I'm hoping that everything I've learned will help make your journeys easier, more enjoyable, productive and impactful because I understand what being a new clinician working in this area means.

The first time I attempted a virtual call I didn't even have a microphone, I hadn't checked I needed one, why would I? No one told me I needed to, and this is exactly the point. If someone doesn't explain or tell us something, how on earth are we supposed to know that a microphone might not be built-in (a webcam, come to that, I've been down that route too!).

DOI: 10.4324/9781003269724-3

It sounds so ridiculous now to think of but, a few years ago I had limited knowledge and I had no one to ask questions of, there was a lot of trial and error until the magic moment where I was on one side of the screen and someone else was on the other (that I could see AND hear at the same time!).

The reality is we all have to start somewhere. At the time of writing, there are no formal routes for new therapists entering the profession to be supported with becoming digital clinicians and to some extent, this makes being a new therapist even harder as they are learning how to be both an SLT and a clinical informatician, and if the training isn't implicit it will feel like two entirely separate roles where never the two shall meet. Some Higher Education Institutions (HEIs) are beginning to weave some elements into the curriculum and have hired digital navigators or digital learning coordinators to support students with remote placements and digital elements of their courses, but there is a lack of emphasis on the skills required of a digital clinician. More on this in Chapter 3 but, first of all, if we know what digital practice is, how can we become a digital practitioner and what is one?

THE TRANSITION: BECOMING A DIGITAL PRACTITIONER

Dispelling the myth that a digital practitioner or clinician only sees people virtually is a good place to start. I've been in many conversations where there is a negativity towards virtual consultations and virtual or remote support in healthcare as it often comes with the assumption that there is a big conspiracy somewhere to replace any and all in person care with a digital service. Whilst digital provision has multiple benefits including providing the potential to support greater efficiency, more joined up services and better transfer of information alongside flexibility and choice of care, it isn't a replacement for in-person appointments. Any care provided should be appropriate for the individual with a focus on their therapeutic targets, functional needs and longterm goals; what works for one person isn't necessarily appropriate for another. New ways of working allow for alternatives in pathways that perhaps were not options previously and now could make the difference between an individual engaging or not. An SLT should always offer choices that are clinically viable and compliant with organisational pathways and processes but beyond this there should be nothing to prevent an SLT from seeing individuals virtually, in-person or 'mixing it up' and doing a combination of the two as a hybrid solution (what some may say is the future of healthcare!). Ultimately whatever is right for the individual is right for the method of delivery and for some, remote sessions offer more flexibility and mean they will engage better in therapy and therefore have better outcomes.

DOI: 10.4324/9781003269724-4

To be a digital practitioner, clinicians need to,

- Be competent and confident in using digital technology as part of their role.
- Provide therapy using digital platforms and mediums.
- Record information using electronic methods and encourage interoperability of information.
- Have an understanding of the importance of data to inform best practices and outcomes for better service provision.
- Be able to create resources using digital programmes.
- Use digital tools to enhance their interventions.
- Safely 'prescribe' and signpost to mobile applications (apps) to support remote monitoring and self-management of a range of conditions.

All of these things do not happen overnight but many of these are facets of an SLT's skill set that they already deploy, they just haven't previously used digital methods to do them or may have but not considered that they were. I for example had been doing digital work for several years but didn't consider myself to be a digital clinician; it was just one element of my skill set and an area I particularly enjoyed doing as I loved to innovate, problem solve and find new ways to do things. Working in digital, or to give it it's proper term, clinical informatics, for me was the perfect fit. It may seem like it happened over night that I went from physical wards to virtual ones but this has evolved over a period of time.

I don't think I had an epiphany moment where I suddenly thought, 'I'm a digital clinician', in fact on occasion I was referred to 'as that SLT that faffs in digital', which made me more determined to show I was most definitely not faffing and I could bring a lot to the digital space because I was good at understanding people and communication was a strong point. On the outside it appeared that I was transitioning rapidly but, for me, this had a been a slow burner that I had been working at for a number of years before I had a real opportunity to use my skills and make a difference. It just happened that it was in the virtual consultation arena and I was able to apply everything I had learned when my organisation needed someone to lead the roll-out of virtual consults across all services and develop a toolkit to enable services to adapt as rapidly as they could in everchanging times and under increasing pressure.

It was a transformation on a size and scale our country has rarely seen, where we suddenly stopped all footfall for in-person appointments and transformed not only services to be virtual but also expected the clinicians delivering the sessions to suddenly be digital practitioners.

Some have embraced it and are thriving on what are often discussed as 'the new ways of working', others are struggling with these changes and have limited experience in or avoided virtual care wherever possible.

What does it take to truly be a digital practitioner? I outlined some of the possible features they might have but they will also be determined, compassionate problem solvers that rise to and thrive on a new challenge. They will seek to maximise each and every opportunity to make the care they deliver the best it can be, but more than this, they will invest time in their colleagues and ensure they have the same knowledge and understanding as themselves in order that the care of the wider service is equitable and everyone is delivering the same level of offer and service regardless of the individual or clinician delivering it.

It isn't easy to achieve and, like all digital transformation, becoming a digital practitioner is part of a process. For those thrust into this place by the pandemic there is a period of reflection and next steps, and for those arriving at the first steps of their journey, where is the best place to start?

The beginning, of course! You wouldn't bake a cake without a recipe, so why would this be any different.

LET'S GET DIGITAL, PART 1! CLINICAL TRAINING OFFERS TO SUPPORT

Throughout the recent pandemic SLTs and wider Allied Health Professionals (AHP) have been quick to unite in their challenges and bring together their experiences, learning and solutions through a range of methods. How many webinars have you attended in the last 24 months for example? This has almost become the norm in rapidly sharing new information, whether you can attend live or not, as if you are registered you will usually receive the link to watch the recording, so even if you are not able to be there you can still be there! There have been webinars to support just about every SLT skill possible, across all the specialities within adult and paediatric services and a common theme across these has been the delivery of virtual consultations. What does this look like? How do you do it? How do we know we are doing it right? In short, who teaches a clinician to become a digital clinician or validates them as competent at conducting a virtual consultation?

The reality is no one. At least this is the case for many professions at present. It is becoming widley recognised that the future of clinicians will be reliant on having adequate digital literacy which will act as a foundation level expected of everyone and will become more specific and targeted as with other clinical competencies.

There are a multitude of networks as well as accredited institutions that individuals can become a member of, but actually signing off competencies specific to disciplines is something that whilst in time is on the horizon is still very much in development (see Chapter 4). Health Education England (HEE)

DOI: 10.4324/9781003269724-5

are also working with NHS Digital, Microsoft and ORCHA to support clinicians with their digital skills and literacy.

Becoming a digital clinician isn't as easy as doing a course on 'how to be a digital clinician'. A little like becoming an SLT, when we qualify it is only the tip of the iceberg, and it is only when we start to hone and develop skills that we develop our specialisms. The same is true of working within informatics as there are so many areas to consider!

There is currently no one national standardised pathway to be certified as a clinician to equip anyone to undertake virtual consultations. The HEE is working with e-learning for health-care (e-lfh) to develop a national digital skills self assessment tool which will enable individuals to be signposted to training specific to their role and support the skills they already have as well as analysing the gaps in knowledge.

Alongside this work, there are further workstreams to create modules specific to virtual consultations happening in partnership with Health Education England, NHS England and NHS Improvement, NHS Digital and e-lfh. This is to support both clinicians providing and individuals receiving care using virtual means, as there will be much more of a level playing field and standardisation. Currently it's very much the luck of the draw. It may be a clinician experienced in providing care virtually or it may be someone very new to the area or who has been reluctant to undertake consulations this way previously. In this instance it isn't the validity of the therapist clinically in question but whether the clinician is confident in using digital tools to provide therapy and how this may impact on the overall delivery and outcomes. Some clinicians have transitioned easily to using virtual consultations within their work and as seen in Chapter 2, may already have familiar skills to enhance their clinical offer. However some clinicians don't have these skills in their tool kit although are still offer-ing virtual consultations even if they do not feel completely equipped to do so. If you were a pupil learning to drive, would you feel comfortable having driving lessons from an instruc-tor who was confident sat in the passenger seat with a clip board but once they got behind the wheel was unsure what happened if they pressed pedals or clicked dials on the dashboard? I imagine the answer is probably no in this context. Why then would it be any different if applied to any other situation where specialist skills are potentially required but not available to everyone to access? At present some healthcare organisations have realised that training to support virtual consultations specifically is needed and so have begun to develop their own packages. The development of support and guidance that the HEE and other national bodies are working to deliver is not just virtual consultation specific training but will encompass broader digital literacy skills to ensure that the future healthcare workforce are equipped with the skills required for the roles they undertake. Long term, clinicians will be competent at the point of qualifying and have a level of digital literacy that will give them sufficient foundations to build their clinical digital skills on.

Your professional body should be your first point of contact for queries about profession-specific information for digital training and for up-to-date clinical informatics information which they may be able to support with or signpost to. Whilst the Royal College of Speech and Language Therapists (RCSLT) has produced a comprehensive guide for telehealth available on their website although at the time of writing they do not offer or endorse any specific informatics training or development specific for SLTs. The information at present is much more general. However there are other sources that may be useful and support your knowledge and understanding of this area.

The Faculty of Clinical Informatics (FCI), which was started in 2017 is well recognised within the clinical informatics community, as is the College of Healthcare Information Management Executives (CHiME), who support a number of initiatives in digital health, as do the Federation of Informatics Professionals (FedIP). All of these carry with them some form of affiliation and membership of varying levels and requirements with intakes at differing times of the year. It is worth understanding what your professional goals are and what you hope to achieve by becoming affiliated with a professional body (what can they do for me, what do they expect of me in return, do I have time?) and whether you can afford the additional payments. Becoming a member of the FCI for example has differing levels of membership but is also linked to FedIP and means clinicians can access materials and forums from their informatics community also. They do not receive further accreditation from FedIP as their professional accreditation is through the FCI but there are benefits to being linked with both and having your network extended further. There are some funded bursaries available to FCI members through the Shuri network, it's not an acronym! For those of you not in the know, Shuri is a character from the Black Panther franchise. Her name was chosen because she is a woman of colour responsible for her country's technological success and was the perfect moniker for a digital health network that supported black and ethnic minority (BAME) women and their allies in health tech. Founded in 2019 by Dr Shera Chok and Sarah Amani, two Chief Clinical Information Officers (CCIO), to support clinicians from diverse backgrounds forge careers in the digital health space by supporting networking, training and development opportunities. Their remit was to raise awareness of the lack of diversity in senior informatics roles within healthcare particularly women of colour because despite 20% of the NHS workforce being from minority ethnic groups and a staggering 77% of these being women, the senior digital roles were limited to just 20 women of colour out of 233 trusts nationally. The Shuri network is a respected, celebrated and enormously supportive community. If you haven't already come across them, they are extremely active on social media and welcome new members so do reach out to them and find out more about their work and the support they offer including shadowing programmes and bursaries for the FCI.

There are also a number of private companies that offer support for clinical skills within virtual consultations specifically. These are not promoted or affiliated with any particular healthcare organisation or clinical body but are an option for those wishing to explore support for their services. This may include a combination of webinar direct, digital skill-based training, as well as role play, soft clinical skill training and how these transfer from in-person to virtual.

COMPLETELY COMPETENT? USING DIGITAL FRAMEWORKS TO DIGITALLY ENABLE CLINICAL WORKFORCES

The importance of workforce competence development is not one which has gone unnoticed, despite the Royal College of Speech and Language Therapists (RCSLT) not yet producing any specific standardised or structured competencies in addition to the current general telehealth guidelines. The guidelines are testament to a community of professionals coming together and sharing their knowledge, experience and desire to make things better at a time of desperation and frustration, however, they have continued to be a well-quoted and valuable resource for SLTs and wider AHPs in the UK and beyond, as much of the guidance is broad based and is not limited to use or applicability in the UK. This is reflected in the fact that many AHP professional bodies have supported Health Education England (HEE) and the Allied Health Profession (AHP) Digital Framework as a sub-framework to the overarching Faculty of Clinical Informatics (FCI) Digital Clinical Framework. It has reduced the need for every royal college to produce their own specific guidance whilst keeping fundamental competencies the same across all 14 professions. Ultimately produced to support clinicians operating within the digital health landscape, forge digital careers and understand their own skill sets to support development and progression, they are a foundation to build upwards from. For some it will be solidifying the basis

DOI: 10.4324/9781003269724-6

of minimal professional expectations, whilst for others it will involve taking the next steps in a digital career.

Both frameworks are based on domains, with the FCI having six domains whilst the AHP Framework has ten. There is an element of overlap but the AHP version published by Health Education England in April 2021 is as it suggests, specific to AHP professions, with the aim being that, as an ongoing piece of work, there will be an interactive framework tailored to each individual profession in time. The framework can be reviewed by searching 'AHP Digital Framework' or using the link in the resources.

These frameworks are available to everyone and I would urge everyone to review them regardless of service or position, particularly the AHP Framework. This will support understanding of what a clinician needs in their digital wheel house and it is expected over time that it will be used as a reference alongside other clinical informatics standards for reviewing clinical digital skills. It may also be something that we see included in Higher Education Institution curriculums as a precursor to the managing, handling and manipulation of patient information using electronic records as well as virtual care.

The ten domains of the framework highlight the breadth of digital and a clinician's role within this landscape. The competencies within each domain are commensurate with a clinician's role and responsibilities, so, the greater the digital role and expectation, the more of the higher-level competencies that are likely to be relevant to you as an individual. This information is briefly presented below to cover the overarching domain titles and the areas within these.

1. General

- Continuing Professional Development (CPD)
- Attitudes and beliefs
- Behaviours
- Foundational and computer skills

2. Data management/clinical informatics

- Information governance
- Cyber security
- Privacy
- Interoperability
- Data evaluation and analytics
- Clinical coding

3. Records assessments and plans

- Structured versus unstructured data in Electronic Health Records (EHR)
- Data capture at point of contact
- EHR system design and modification

4. Transfer of Care

- Risks
- Data sharing
- Personalised care

5. Medicine management and optimisation

- E-prescription
- Automated dispensing
- Independent prescribing
- Patient Group Directions (PGDs)/Patient Specific Directions (PSDs)
- Electronic Medicines Optimisation Pathway (EMOPs)

6. Orders and results management

- Diagnostics/screening monitoring
- Pathology/laboratory medical imaging
- viewing, sharing and storing data
- Artificial Intelligence (AI) and Machine Learning (ML)

7. Assets resource optimisation

- Organisation
- Personal

8. Decision support

- Automated evidence-based guidelines with systems
- Associated AI and ML
- Risks and bias
- Professional responsibility

9. Digital therapeutics

- Clinically assured health information
- Remote care
- Health apps and devices
- Other patient-facing technologies

10. Meta-competencies

- Leadership
- Strategy
- Quality improvement and research
- Change management
- Governance

In respect of virtual consultations specifically as highlighted in Chapter 3, there is yet to be anything nationally formalised or standardised by NHS England or by Health Education England, but it is an area that is being addressed at the time of writing by national bodies as it has been raised in acknowledgement of the discussions around workforce development and equipping clinicians with the appropriate skills and knowledge. At present, the closest thing available has been produced by NHS England and Health Education England and is part of what is a 'total triage' packge which consists of seven separate modules with a number of videos via the e-lfh platform. It is an update of an earlier iteration which was a report produced in early Covid-19, supported by a number of YouTube videos. It is primarily for General Practitioners and primary care so is structured around very primary care specific scenarios and contexts. Some information is relatable and transferable but not all of it is relevant or applicable. At the time of writing it also isn't as yet a fully realised training package but work to develop aspects of this to make relevant for further clinical groups is underway in order that it can be assigned to clinicians or associate clinicians to prepare for undertaking virtual consultation in secondary, community or social care settings. Once this offer is developed it will hopefully be one that encompasses clinicians across all levels of healthcare and provides both a solid foundation for competency, as well as the potential to act as a refresher to boost confidence. This may be useful after a period of not practising, for example returning from a leave of absence, maternity or ill health and allow a clinician to familiarise themselves with the premise of virtual working, covering safety, security, responsibilities and practicalities, as well as transferable clinical skills relevant to virtual delivery.

DIGITAL CONFIDENCE: WHAT DOES THIS MEAN IN A CLINICAL CONTEXT?

You can't see it or touch it, so how do you know if you or someone else has it? Can it be measured? Unlike competencies which can be measured, tested and recorded, building confidence comes from personal experience, perspective and ability to transfer clinical skills from one scenario to another. Without a doubt, some people will find this easier than others to realise, but how do you build confidence in a new skill?

PRACTICE HELPS!

It may sound like the most patronising thing to say in the known world but it really can make a huge amount of difference to build your confidence by familiarising yourself with tools, routines, objectives and aims and delivering your sessions in an alternative way. Having the opportunity to practise can make that daunting first session seem less daunting because you are reducing the unknowns from the equation. As a neurodiverse person the more places or times I can do this the better, as I can have elevated anxiety about new situations. I may not be alone in this feeling, and if there are other clinicians feeling like this then imagine how many members of the public that may be waiting for therapy could be experiencing similar situations. Section 2 has a lot of information about how to prepare someone for a virtual consultation and the same principles are equally applicable to us as clinicians; just because we are the professionals doesn't mean we don't get spooked or scared. Actually this can be far from it, as we often feel

DOI: 10.4324/9781003269724-7

a clinical responsibility to ensure that what we deliver is the best it can be, and to do so is to put our own personal fears and experiences aside, when perhaps we can harness these emotions and experiences to inform how those we care for may be feeling, while also validating that it is perfectly normal to feel that way in a new situation ourselves.

USE YOUR COLLEAGUES

When I say use them, I don't mean start asking them if they will buy you a coffee every Friday, promise to pay them back and never have your wallet with you, I mean use them to help you build your confidence. Ask them to test your knowledge and skills, mock up a test scenario and act out a role play and ask them for tips or ideas to improve your delivery. Don't be afraid to make notes and practice again. Use the information to record a personalised video or practice recording yourself delivering a session: can you find all the buttons you need to, can you screen share, does your presentation play (with the audio?), can you see yourself, hear yourself, is the connection stable?

Rule all the techy bits out and then focus on your clinical delivery. Are you getting in all the information you usually would? It might help to boost your confidence by writing a short script for each section as segue into the next section and ensuring you keep to time. The beauty about virtual delivery is no one can see what is on the desk in front of you, so if you need a few flashcards or post-it-notes as prompts, use them until you feel comfortable, if you ever saw the other side of my screen you'd think my laptop had post-it-note plague!

TOP TIP: Stick your post it notes down one side of the screen (across the top risks blocking the camera). I pull them off as I complete a prompt, it's like my own mini visual timetable!

Your prompts might include quick references to,

- Introduce yourself.
- Conduct security checks (see Section 2).
- Introduce the session objectives and refer back to them as needed.
- Consider any assessments (formal/informal) that need to be undertaken.
- Is there any recap or feedback from previous session that needs to be given?
- Set goals.
- Prompt the person you are delivering the session to when they have a few minutes left to enable you to round up the session and provide you with a natural route to shut down the consultation.
- Plan next steps for intervention.
- Book an appointment if possible, advise if they will be sent the information and don't forget to record this.
- Physically shut down the session (see Section 2 for how to make sure you have safely logged out).

As with becoming a digital practitioner the confidence to be one comes with time. The first in-person session we do can be nerve-racking but exciting as we have prepared and practised, planned resources, researched everything we can about the case history and want to be the best we can. Nothing is different in delivering a digital session, channel any nervous energy and know that if you can survive an in-person appointment you can survive a virtual one because it's the same skills, same therapy, but with a different method of delivery.

A NEW WAY OF PRACTISING OR JUST PRACTISING A NEW WAY?

My honest opinion (for what it's worth) is we aren't reinventing the wheel and we actually don't need to. We are taking what we already do as flexible, adaptable and able clinicians and delivering therapy simply using a different method … if you read Chapter 5 that won't be any great shock!

We aren't suddenly inherently different as clinicians just because there is a screen between us and the other person (or group), we are just using the skills we have creatively and tuning ourselves into a different delivery method.

The differences are,

- We have to be more aware of security and sharing information that doesn't put us or those we care for at risk.
- We need to be confident in using a computer and navigating between browsers and screens (and knowing the difference between the two – Section 2 can help!).
- We have to multitask more than usual moving between screens (the virtual consultation and the person's health record).
- The assessments we use might be in a different format.
- The place we write our notes might be different.
- The reports we write might be in a different format or shared in a different way using digital tools.

The similarities are,

- We are the same person and the therapy we are providing is the same.

DOI: 10.4324/9781003269724-8

- The assessments we use are the same.
- The outcome measures are the same.
- The professionals we refer to are the same.
- The reports we write are the same.
- The goals we strive for are the same.
- The professionalism we display is the same.
- The clinical skills we apply are the same.

Overall the similarities outweigh the differences, indicating that rather than it being a new way of practising we are just practising in a new way using all the skills we already have and blending them with a few new skills that we may not have used in a clinical setting previously but may be familiar within our personal lives, such as multitasking as we manage banking or utility bills or increasing our cyber security skills as we indulge in online shopping.

We may still be adapting to these newer ways of working, or, for some who are newly entering the profession, encountering the scenarios and skills for the first time, but we are still learning and developing these skills together. There were no rules or guidance in place prior to Covid-19, and whilst at times it has been frustrating, challenging and even concerning that more structured guidance or competency frameworks were not in place, no one was prepared for the onslaught that the pandemic brought. Yes, the NHS Long Term Plan mapped out this as a goal, but it was based on a ten-year plan and that was rapidly cut short. So perhaps it's fortunate that we are now in a position where we can actually inform that training and guidance alongside the future of curriculums for new therapists entering the profession through Higher Education or Apprenticeship programmes? We have the ability to use our real life experience and advise what actually happens on the 'shop floor' and inform guidance that can be impactful, useful and relevant instead of something we tick off and never refer to again. Training should be a living part of what we do, or how is it relevant?

Virtual strikes fear in many people I've spoken to and I do understand where this is from, a fear of change (I hate change), of something being outside of your control, of not being explained to, of not being supported, of not being listened to when ideas are shared or warnings that it won't work because x, y, z happens in real life, but virtually different doesn't mean virtually impossible.

I hope it can mean that we embrace a new way of working, one that is alternative, flexible, adaptable and offers dignity and promotes independence of choice in healthcare.

Virtual consultations will not be appropriate for all patients and not all people will want them, some will want them where it's not clinically viable, some will want them but digital exclusion is a factor and increases the possibility of health inequality and should be something considered when discussing options with the individual (is there any way this can be mitigated, can the service/organisation/charity support with device/data/training to enable someone to participate using virtual consultations if they want to and if it is viable).

We as clinicians ultimately should make an informed decision based on the service we work in and the pathways available, clinical appropriateness and individual choice about their healthcare because we aren't different, we are just doing what we would have done if they had been in-person. Digital is an enabler, let it enable.

A Digital Stage!

Before I trained as a speech and language therapist my first love was the stage. So it seems strange to have gone full circle and be considering what we do in therapy in theatrical terms. Every time I've done a virtual consultation I have this strange feeling I'm in a bizarre YouTube video! Quite who would want to like and subscribe to that channel I do not know, but it makes me smile and somehow lessens my anxiety and fear if I view it as another conversation with someone I know well.

The first time I heard the term 'virtual platform' the image was people stood waiting for something at a station! So what is a platform if it isn't somewhere to catch the 7am from St Pancras on a Monday morning? In simple terms, the platform that we use to deliver virtual care is a web- or app-based piece of technology that allows secure video calls to be made between clinicians and patients. The method we use may differ, but the skills we use are largely the same, and many of the major players of virtual consultation platforms in digital health use similar functions and operate in a way that could be a copy and paste of another with a different branding meaning that for users that can provide a very similar experience and make it a little easier to navigate if your organisation uses different platforms to offer these services. Now we are further in the virtual revolution than from the outset of the pandemic, many organisations have tested the market and have begun to commit to one solution rather than multiple, realising that for the public it is much better to have a single a streamlined and simplified user experience (UX) whilst from a clinical systems perspective it is also easier.

Over the course of the pandemic it felt like a new solution was being built and released onto the market daily. From huge industry leaders and national partnerships like that of

26

DOI: 10.4324/9781003269724-9

Microsoft and the NHS, to smaller developments from global distributors breaking into the healthcare market in the UK having been frontrunners in other continents for decades.

The UK was 'behind the front door' as the saying goes when it came to virtual consultations, as many other countries had been delivering virtual care for long periods, including Scotland. Other countries, including America, Australia, Canada and Greece had been using virtual consultations for a number of years in speech and language therapy, so the concept was not a new one to many in these localities and business was very much as usual. The level of complexity and innovation was on a scale I hadn't anticipated, having both researched and collaborated with clinicians working at the other side of the globe. One such example was of clinicians working to support patients more than 150 miles away from a clinic in Texas, working with immigrant communities where new stomas had led to complexities, emergency department admissions and increased infant mortality due to poor tracheostomy care with families failing to return for follow up appointments. The telehealth service enabled families to be supported and trained, minimising risks and increasing outcomes for the child (Moreno and Peck, 2020). Virtual can be an amazing tool when used effectively and has also proved a useful solution for remote communities where regular clinicians are not always available. In these instances it means contact can be maintained for therapeutic purposes even so children in remote communities can be supported effectively by clinicians and their parents. Following the initial pilot a teacher reported 'that telehealth is a great option for those rural areas'. So despite the intermittent internet challenges it was felt that this method demonstrated the possibility to 'enable widespread implementation of telerehabilitation services into rural schools' (Bradford et al., 2018), if there's a signal there's a way and a remote possibility

Choosing a platform may not be something you are able to do as often it is determined by the organisation you are working within and the contract they are aligned to. Until recently, many NHS organisations had funded access to Attend Anywhere, which was rolled out nationally almost overnight during the first few weeks of the pandemic to limit the 'whatever works' mindset that had the potential to cause security breaches and further complications from an information governance perspective. Now this support has ended at a national level, NHS organisations are required to make their own arrangements for a virtual consultation platform. For this reason there may be more variation across some geographical areas than others. For some organisations who have been keen to streamline systems already in place, they have used this change as an opportunity to consider utilising the video consultation ability of Microsoft (MS) Teams, alongside other functions, the Office 365 and suite of MS Teams tools functions offers in terms of interoperability across an organisation or even more widely into an Integrated Care System (ICS). Whereas others have preferred to stay with legacy systems they are familiar with and consider migrating to alternate platforms for the long term at a later date.

There are no right and wrong answers, they are answerable to themselves, their digital strategy and agendas but also need to account for their rationale and decision making in their funding bids, so making convincing statements can be difficult and it is worth bearing in mind when you are desperate for your setting to use a particular platform and you keep getting told no … there is usually a good reason why.

It may be funding related, it may be security, information governance (IG) localised or system-wide agreements, but ask if you are unsure. The IG or clinical safety team can be really helpful in these instances, as more often than not a platform isn't approved because there is an IG concern or a digital clinical assurance concern that hasn't been addressed by the supplier and the organisation quite rightly isn't willing to put its staff or the public at risk simply because 'everyone uses X platform for the Saturday night quiz'.

For those not in NHS settings who may have more influence over the platform, it may be worth reviewing the RCSLT telehealth guidance as there is a comprehensive guide to platforms within this, and although it may not have every update (there are updates happening all the time so it's almost impossible to keep up) it gives an overview of the main platforms and some of the lesser-known platforms that may be viable options in private sector settings.

Some top tips to consider when using a platform, whether one used by an organisation or if you are supporting a procurement of your own,

- Does it support more than one person on a call, i.e. can you add more people in a useful feature for hosting Multi Disciplinary Team (MDTs)?
- Does it have a chat function?
- Can you signpost at the end of the session to feedback or therapy information via a link? – not a deal breaker, but can be useful rather than having to send a further message or email with a link in it if they are auto-directed.
- How many people does it support? – considering group therapy, some only consistently support up to 4 people (i.e it gets a little bit unstable if you start bringing on the whole team plus various relatives) which isn't great if you have a group of 12!
- Can you screen share?
- Does it have a chat function? – useful if the video or microphone connection is lost to communicate and revert to another mode or give directions.
- Can you share attachments/upload files?
- Does it have captions or dynamic transcriptions? Can you keep a record of these and upload to the inidividuals health record or share with them if the request?
- Does it record? Do you need to, where would you you store it after? (Does your organisation allow this? – see Section 2.)

If you are having difficulty with the practicality of using a platform, ask a colleague, and if they don't have the answer, log a job with IT for the IT trainers. They may have a manual they can email or that is available on the organisation's intranet or they may arrange either a 1:1 or session for the service to train you up. No question is a silly one if you don't have the answer and worry breeds a lack of confidence and fear. If we can reduce the fear of a situation then the likelihood is we can be more confident about using the platform to deliver therapy and may, in time, feel confident to support others.

8

ARE DIGITAL CLINICS DIFFERENT? WHAT ARE THEY AND HOW ARE THEY IMPLEMENTED?

The only difference is that they are not in a physical setting. Everything else is as you would expect it to be if they were run in-person. Appointments are booked and managed, people attend (virtually), caseloads are managed accordingly and outcomes are updated and monitored.

They can be more tiring for the clinician in relation to the physical and mental exertion required to manage a whole clinic list of just virtual appointments versus being able to stretch your legs to collect someone from a waiting room or pop down the hall to a classroom if you are in an educational setting. The danger is that we don't take the rest and breaks that we would if we were in a workplace, no one pops by your desk with a cup of tea and a biscuit or asks if you want a walk around the grounds at lunch time to get some fresh air. If you are disciplined, you may have found ways of building some of these self-care elements into your day and Section 4 has some tips for how you can balance your well-being alongside virtual working.

First and foremost a digital clinic will have a clinic list in exactly the same way an in-person one does.

It will also typically be built around a particular condition so you already have an awareness of what to expect in that clinic, be it phonology, dysfluency, aphasia or voice disorders.

The assessments, interventions and activities will be the same as you would have prepared for in-person therapy. The difference in a digital clinic, as with the similarities and differences presented in Chapter 2, will be that the format of these

DOI: 10.4324/9781003269724-10

may be electronic versions rather than paper-based, so they are shareable on screen and can be uploaded into electronic records with relative ease as a PDF.

Digital clinic management versus traditional or in-person clinics, will (or should be) similar in terms of decisions made about each individual as these will still influence waiting lists across the wider service, impacting other aspects of caseload management. For example, this may include the length of time an individual is waiting to be seen, discharge rates and number of episodes of care as well as considering those who consistently do not attend and if someone else could benefit by being offered their place for therapy.

It's useful to collate data on these areas of digital clinics particularly around rates of discharge to compare efficacy and appropriacy, as if a patient is actually having more appointments over a longer period of time, digital care may not be the most clinically appropriate for them or the condition they have.

It could be that hybrid options are also a consideration and are an option that some services and clinicians are moving towards for a number of reasons. To reduce screen fatigue, to maximise clinical efficacy and to maximise service efficiency. This means that a clinician may see a combination of both video, telephone and face-to-face patients within a single clinic as long as the service is equipped to allow this way of working.

Another consideration is having a number of individuals all working on the same therapy goals in tandem, could digital clinics be used to provide therapy for them all in one session rather than all separately? This has the benefit of peer support and encouragement, networking for individuals who have similar experiences and reducing waiting lists by seeing multiple numbers rather than one at a time, enabling more people to be seen in a shorter time scale.

The management of clinics using digital tools are as much an important consideration as the delivery of the clinic itself. It may be worth discussing with the team you work in what elements of clinic management are digitised already, and whether there are others which could be brought in to increase efficiency, such as automating further processes (reminders, updates, follow-up appointment emails); could reports be sent digitally, except where specifically asked for a paper copy to reduce both carbon footprint and increase amount of information being shared digitally?

Could this same information be shared or flagged with all healthcare professionals working with that individual via a central record?

The internet has multiple examples of digital clinics, either 1:1 or in groups across a range of speech and language therapy specialities, where interventions have worked really well such as the Lee Silverman Voice Therapy Programme, voice disorders, phonology, language delays and disorders and social communication, including the assessment of autism using online tools.

Good digital transformation doesn't have to mean big changes, it could be the small changes that make a big difference!

VIRTUAL VOICES! SHARING BEST PRACTICE AND RESOURCES

You may have already started collating a file of information on your computer of handy websites, useful app names, top tips for how-to guides or references to read at an as yet unidentified date because there aren't enough hours in the day to do virtual clinics, make the bed, wash your hair and cook something other than beans on toast maybe? You may even have come up with your own ideas for therapy based on experiences you have had delivering sessions, workshopping new ideas in your team or creating new resources for your caseload. Think of all that lovely information and learning we could share across our community! If you as just one person reading this has got something to share, imagine how many others may have something they may be able to share, too. A whole electronic encyclopaedia of telehealth information that, instead of sitting on someone's computer waiting to be read, could be used by someone on the other side of the country to help a child master 'S' clusters using a new digital resource that has been shared or supported a person rehabilitating after a stroke with word-finding difficulties and has some brilliant app recommendations.

If you have a problem, chances are someone has a solution, maybe unknowingly, but I would be confident that if they recognise what they have may be helpful they would be willing to share. This being the case, I'd like to encourage sharing of resources far and wide across social media. The SLT and digital AHP community, both in the UK and beyond, are particularly active on Twitter:

DOI: 10.4324/9781003269724-11

Speechie Chat @SpeechChat
WeSpeechies @wespeechies
Dr Abi Roper @abracabadger
SLTs of Colour @OfSlts
On the Same Team @SLTsSameTeam
Digital AHP Network @NetworkAhp
Shuri Network @NetworkShuri

So let's grow our community, add the #remotelyresources when you share or search for resources and if you tag me @RemotelyPossib1 I will also share your replies and resources. So let's unite our virtual voices and grow our remote resources to support each other as we continue our journeys as digital practitioners.

THE REMOTE
RULES

10

THE BIG CLICK ON: BEFORE A REMOTE CONSULTATION

This chapter will prepare you to prepare. Making clear the considerations that you should make before undertaking a session, whether it be the first, fiftieth or five hundredth, the same processes are applicable for the safety of the person and protection of the clinician undertaking.

By breaking the process down and reviewing what preparation will make for a session that's safe, productive and efficient we can ensure no stone is left unturned. In order to use technology to support a person's needs there are multiple considerations and factors to evidence in order to be both compliant and considered a success. Not only relative to the therapy but in achieving service user outcomes, broader service delivery requirements, information governance, digital clinical patient safety and bringing all these together to meet the digital first aim of the NHS Long Term Plan.

RECEIVING A REFERRAL

Globally, many speech and language services, across both adults and paediatric within private and public sectors, offer a self-referral process. Meaning that an individual, parent or caregiver with swallowing and/or communication symptoms or problems can refer themselves to an appropriate service directly without having to wait to seek the opinion of a general practitioner (GP), Ear Nose and Throat (ENT) specialist, audiologist, health visitor, school nurse or other healthcare professional in order to be triaged by a speech and language therapist/pathologist (SLT/SLP). Historically the self-referral process may have included multiple ways of a service user being able to refer in, including fax and email as well as standard telephone referrals with completion of paper forms. With technology being ever more adopted to enhance all engagement with services, the introduction of electronic processes and apps are being used to collate and support self-management of personal healthcare records and encourage individuals to have responsibility and autonomy for their own healthcare management.

The use of applications, commonly known as apps, as well as digitised self-referrals embedded on external organisations websites, allows for a service user to request a referral directly through a secure and approved method of service engagement. This serves to streamline the referral process with a focus on encouraging patients to have more responsibility and ownership in their healthcare management and is a significant driver of the wider, long-term agendas as well as the current response to mitigating a number of inequalities of care alongside reducing waiting times.

If an app is not in use in your organisation or practice, it is easy to create a self-referral form and request the Uniform Resource Locator (URL), more familiar as the URL or the address of a webpage. This is posted on your services webpage on the organisational website for individuals to have access to referring in this way. The same URL can be used to create a Quick Response or QR code. They look like square barcodes and they are capable of holding a lot of data. They are like a fingerprint for a website or webpage and it's easier than you may think to create one. The easiest way is,

- To use your preferred search engine to search for 'Free QR code generator'. There are several that will come up and are all relatively straightforward to use.
- Type in the URL where prompted and the site will generate a QR code for you.
- You will be given the option to download the image, which you can then add to any communications sent to individuals.

- Always check the QR code works by testing it out before you use it for mass communication. You can do this by scanning the QR code using your mobile phone camera. If it is working correctly it will bring up the website or web-page name you are directing to and, when clicked on, will take you to it. See resources for more information on how to generate a QR code.

In addition to supporting self-referral, QR codes can also be used for promotion of the service in public areas (posters on corridors, notice boards and information areas) within an organisation or added to publications for advertising and awareness purposes.

A benefit of using electronic methods in addition to driving referrals forward and offering service users options to engage and manage their care, by having a central inbox which is managed by appropriate staff, the service can monitor the frequency, volume and flow of referrals enabling efficient data provision for service audits and evaluation.

TOP TIP: It is highly useful to identify in an initial referral whether a service user is equipped, eager and willing to engage in video consultations, in the absence of administrative support or other pathways such as the use of virtual receptionists that can support individuals with the technical aspects of engagement. As time is limited during appointments and should be focussed on therapy, it removes an additional factor for clinicians if it has been established pre-appointment, not only if a patient is willing to engage but actually that they have appropriate infrastructure, including stable internet, data, hardware (a tablet, smartphone, laptop or desktop with webcam and microphone) before being able to offer an initial appointment.

This not only establishes whether a virtual consultation is a viable method to arrange for a particular individual based on what they do have access to, but it has the potential to highlight any barriers to engagement that may prevent or impact virtual care being a possibility and gives time to resolve these ahead of the session. These may include access to equipment, data and the affordability of this, context and privacy of setting for the appointment, accessibility factors physically, emotionally and cognitively. Protected characteristics (Equality Act, 2010) and engagement of virtual consultations are of particular relevance when considering health inequalities and how we can mitigate against these when offering care using digital pathways.

Once established if these are available, the process of booking and how this might differ to in-person appointments is the next stage of preparation.

BOOKING APPOINTMENTS

In the same way we would book an in-person appointment, a video consultation should be treated and booked (wherever possible) using processes which are similar. This also means a virtual appointment should be subject to the same process as a Did Not Attend (DNA), adhering to the same policy that would apply if it was an in-person format. A virtual appointment for both service user and service should be viewed with the same level of significance because your time as a clinician is still valuable and accounted for, regardless of how the session is being delivered.

In all aspects of the video consultation pathway, aim to replicate as much of the service delivery model from in-person delivery as possible. This is effectively to map one type of delivery method against the other, aiming for an equitable model of care, delivering wherever possible the same high-quality care, assessment and management as would be received if a service user was attending a setting as an outpatient.

For example, offering a virtual appointment to a service user may be undertaken in several ways. They may receive a letter in the post or, increasingly, as a letter within an email or SMS as an attachment or link. The letter should include,

1. Date and time. It may be helpful to include wording advising to encourage individuals to book the date and time and indicate that the appointment will be treated as a standard appointment with service policy regarding nonattendance whether the appointment is clinic-based or virtually delivered.

2. Depending on the platform you are using, either,

   - Include the link if generated at the time of booking appointment.
   - Highlight that closer to their appointment time (include timescales if known, i.e. one day before, one hour before etc.) that they will receive a link to join the consultation.

This is one example of translating a face-to-face appointment into a digital alternative. Other possibilities include residential settings, education and both primary and acute care settings. It can be helpful to map out the current process if not already available and review what amends need to be included for digital pathways as with the above example.

IMPORTANT: Ensure that you have used the usual booking process using the Electronic Patient Record (EPR) system if your organisation uses one. Use the appropriate coding so that the service is paid accordingly for the session. This means using the appropriate contact method for recording in the services diary or booking system. This may be the wording, icon or both, so it is wise to familiarise yourself with the requirements of your own organisation to ensure you are consistent and accurate in how virtual consultations are being booked and appearing within clinical systems (e.g. can you record video appointments and phone appointments under separate codes/options, or is it 'virtual' for either?). Another factor when considering booking an appointment alongside coding is cost. At present within the NHS, there is no standardised differentiation between the cost of an in-person session or a virtual consultation. This is the same for missed appointments.

For independent practice you must draw on your policy for cancellations and rebooking of in-person and consider if you will apply the same processes also. For an equivalent offer, plus simplicity of policy and pricing structures, consider having the same open and clear policy for the booking and cancellation of video/phone consultations.

As with SMS, it is imperative to have all communications sent and received by a generic and approved inbox. For NHS Mail users a quick and easy way to ensure security in your emails will be discussed in more detail in the next chapter. For other organisations, please ensure the mail tenant you use is secure and has end-to-end encryption to protect any information shared between yourself and the service user.

11

VIRTUAL VIRGINS

It's all well and good getting the referral sorted, booking a date and sending out a link, but what if the service users are virtual virgins?

We've all been there and worn that hat and can therefore reflect with renewed digital confidence, 'if only we knew then what we know now', so perhaps it is beneficial to use this thought process to prepare others for their first forays into virtual consultations and ensure we have covered every base we can in doing so. The primary one of these being the supporting user guides for whichever platform is the stage for your interaction.

Consider the who, what, where, when and how (it's often a useful way of identifying user, purpose, timing and method).

WHO DO YOU NEED TO SEND THE INFORMATION TO?

If a child has been referred then it will likely be an individual with parental responsibility, but you may also want to share a version with children and/or young people to explain the process and even outline the need for them to support 'grown ups' or adults as even very young children can find their way around an iPad and a smartphone!

If the service user is a care home resident, will you send the information to the care home as well as a named relative or Lasting Power of Attorney (LPA) in case they want to join the session or just need to be kept in the loop?

The audience will have an impact on WHAT you send.

WHAT ARE YOU GOING TO SEND? MAKING INFORMATION ACCESSIBLE AND INCLUSIVE

Is the standard information and user guide suitable for the intended service user, cohort or organisation, or does an accessible version need to be created for a service user? This could be bespoke in the first instance, but it's pretty much a guarantee if one service user needs a particular format then another will, be that in your own service or somewhere else in the world. Will it be a written guide or an alternative format such as an animated video resource on YouTube or embedded on your organisation or practice's website? Some platforms have already produced 'how to guides' in this format, whilst for others you may need to ask the platform supplier to create one or even ask your internal departments for an organisation-specific 'how-to guide'. This can be helpful on a number of levels as there is the additional feature of familiarity as it is someone from a trusted source sharing the information.

This highlights the importance of sharing and shouting about resources, so that, be it your work or the work of others, if you have found and used something that's been really helpful, it can be used to support service users near and far. After all, there's no point in having a great resource if only you know about it!

TOP TIP: If you are creating accessible resources you will be happy to share, don't forget to make them editable, such as adaptable background colour for visual comfort in dyslexic service users. You can always ask that you are referenced or acknowledged if it is something you are really passionate about. You could create a bank of documents if you are a prolific resource maker and host them on your own online drive to share them in the RCSLT Telehealth Forum or the equivalent, for example in Speech Pathology Australia (SPA) or American Speech and Hearing Association (ASHA) as well as sharing using the #remotelyresources on Twitter with the SLT community for others to use.

In the same vein, there's no harm in asking if the community of SLT/SLPs has anything you can magpie and repurpose, even if it was for another platform in the first place, typically the principles are the same. (See resources for examples of user guides for style, content and accessibility, including animation format.)

WHY ARE YOU SENDING IT?

Is it to give them a whistle stop overview, an in-depth 'how-to guide', or a quick reference guide to have to hand as a prompt. This interlinks with WHAT as the purpose, as well as the person, may define the reason it's being sent.

For example, it might be in the format of any number of these,

- One-page written guide.
- One-page, picture-based guide.
- Infographic with easy read icons and bespoke colours.
- In-depth leaflet or brochure.
- A corporate or bespoke animation.

WHEN ARE YOU SENDING IT?

Think about when you are sending the information out to have the most impact. Consider how far in advance the appointment has been booked to guide whether sending it at the time of booking is most appropriate or scheduling a reminder to send a few days before so the information is fresh in the service user's mind and they are less likely to mislay the information.

HOW ARE YOU SENDING IT?

It might be useful to consider how the appointment was booked and acknowledged with the service user as this may be their preferred method of receiving and interacting with information.

Some service users may prefer to have a 'hard copy', otherwise known as a paper copy received in the post. Where this is the case it can be encouraged or advocated that you will send an SMS or email to a registered and validated number or email address with the relevant information.

You may want to consider using the 'digital by default' approach first and only send hard copies if specifically requested, thus supporting paperless or paperlite processes.

SMS: Some platforms and EPRs will allow you to attach documents to an SMS such as photographs, PDFs or MS Word files. It will allow the person to open and view these on their device. There are no hard and fast rules for how to send information as long as it is via an approved process that is secure and you may find that even within a single organisation there are different pathways for sharing, although informal evaluation suggests that SMS is a preferred method by many persons as it doesn't require them to open up other devices (some people choose not to have their emails on their phones).

As with attachments, copy and pasting hyperlinks or URLs for animations, embedded documents, etc. can easily be inserted via this method. Depending on the messaging and push system used, there may be a limited word count so it may help to use a template for wording to ensure service information is highlighted for security and reassurance as well as including the information. You could ask for a reply to validate that they have received it. The message will appear from your organisation when the person receives it if it is a platform that integrates with the NHS spine for the public sector or with a personal e-rostering or scheduling system for the private sector. You should not send communications to a service user from a personal mobile unless it is for exclusive work use, so as to not put your own information at risk as service users may then use this to contact you inappropriately out of your working hours and lead to information governance breaches as it will not be a secure or encrypted service if it is a personal network.

Typically the services are internet-based and use a centralised number to push the notifications from. This service is secure.

EMAIL: This is basically a replica of the SMS process but, of course, using a service user's email address and if a service user has expressed this is their preferred method, documents and links can be attached and embedded in the same way as an SMS (just make sure you are using an encrypted email).

For NHS Mail users, although the NHS Mail server is secure, it is not always possible to know that the individual or organisation with whom the information is being shared is also secure. There are a number of secure email addresses that are considered safe and there are encryption softwares that some organisations may use when sending confidential information. However, an individual or private organisation may have a non-secure domain but may still want or need to share information with clinical services. This means that, without password encryption or other security measures, the information shared could be accessed by unintended recipients.

A quick and easy method of mitigating against this is to create a secure email chain by using the NHS Mail account. By sending and receiving an email from and to an NHS Mail account it creates a secure chain which will enable the sender to share information securely. For more tips on attachments, visit Section 3 – Getting Attached.

EXAMPLE OF WHO, WHAT, WHEN AND HOW

SCENARIO A: PARENT AND FIVE-YEAR-OLD GIRL

They have never had a virtual consultation before and the parent is very anxious that their daughter won't sit still during the session because she is at home and might be distracted.

WHO

- A parent
- Five-year-old child

WHAT

- The link to join the session.
- A parent may benefit from a quick written user guide with tips for keeping a child occupied during the session

reassuring them that it doesn't matter if they are distracted, it will still be a very useful session to have.

- The child may find it easier to watch a short animation talking them through the process or read a story about another child that has had the same sort of appointment – shared experiences. There is a platform agnostic video and resources; now available on the National Video Consultation page via NHS Futures. **Please be aware you will need to register if not already and request to join the workspace, Video consultations for NHS secondary care providers – NHSFutures Collaboration Platform**.

TOP TIP: It may be helpful to include a short activity that the child can do in preparation to act as an ice-breaker, such as,

- Ask them to bring a cuddly toy to introduce (this can be a useful vehicle for engagement and language too!).
- Make a list of five things they like to do.
- Draw a picture of their family to share (this can also be used as part of the identity-check process, i.e. 'who's in the house today?').

WHY

- The parent needs to know how to log on and join a call, trouble shoot etc.
- The child needs to be reassured of what will happen, how long it will take, who they might see and what they and their 'grown up' might be expected to do in the session.

WHEN

You may opt to send this out at the time of the booking for the parent and a few days ahead for the child, or both at the same time and send a check-in message a few days ahead of the appointment to remind the parent to watch the animation with the child, allowing time for them to get in touch prior to the session if the child has any questions.

HOW

The most obvious process would be to send out the link and information for the session using the same method. Typically this will be directly to the service user via email or SMS.

However, there may be alternate methods of signposting that you could consider. These will depend on what is available within your organisation but are worthwhile considering as there may be a particular option you want to make available within your service.

- URL to a direct website.
- Organisation website with embedded video.
- Organisation website with downloadable user guides/ information resources in varying formats for different service user groups. This option will:
  o Allow you to signpost the service user/users to relevant information.
  o Afford the service user accountability in self-managing an element of their own care in following the advice to read information as well as selecting the most appropriate format for themselves.

Having already established a two-way interaction with the service user through email and or SMS, you are already enabling and empowering them to be autonomously involved in the telehealth process as well as fulfilling duty of care in regard to appropriate and accessible engagement and information.

IMPORTANT: Don't forget that it is imperative to have all communications *sent and received* by a central (sometimes called generic) and approved inbox within your service via a secure mail tenant with end-to-end encryption. This is to protect any information shared between yourself and the service user.

12

TESTING, TESTING

TESTING EQUIPMENT

Everything is in place for a session, but you join the call and the service user can't hear you! Panic fills you and you flap about, clicking buttons, leaving and joining the call in an attempt to rectify in line with the platform's own troubleshooting advice. Although there is no guarantee this won't happen every now and again for reasons known only to device demons, there are a number of ways to reduce the chances, and it's the simple act of testing. The platform you are using may run a check for you as you initiate the call.

- Test camera – make sure your camera is on, obvious but necessary and, for most platforms, the most obvious way is if you can see yourself on screen!
- Test microphone – make sure your microphone is on so that the service user can hear you but also ensure that the volume is turned up sufficiently for you to hear the others on the call.

To check volume is turned up, locate the speaker icon, which is usually on the bottom toolbar of the laptop or desktop and double click to slide to the desired volume. Alternatively, this may just be a quick click of the volume buttons on a tablet or smartphone if you are conducting a session in this way.

DOI: 10.4324/9781003269724-15

LET'S GET DIGITAL, PART 2: PREPARING SERVICE USERS FOR CHANGE

Clinicians being prepared and 'clicked on' for action is only half of the preparation. As with in-person therapy or consultations, a service user must also be fully on board with a process, not just the practical preparation but also the psychological. A service user that is prepared for what to expect as much as what is expected, will be able to engage more successfully, leading to therapeutic outcomes with purpose.

So how do we as clinicians ensure we are bringing our service users with us on the digital journey? I intend this to be a very practical guide to support clinicians setting up digital clinics, so I will address the core elements and link to relevant resources and guidance as well as considerations for how to create and develop them.

The RCSLT Telehealth Guidelines, as with many aspects of this guidance, are a mine of useful information and advice, and have examples of such resources which may be useful to review as part of this element of the process. I of course acknowledge that each service will have different service users' needs to consider dependent on provision but, regardless of this, nationally, we should be aiming to ensure all information is accessible and inclusive from the outset. Not only is this integral to successful communication at all levels with those we are caring for and supporting, but preparation in advance will enhance timely and efficient support for all service users. Accessible material being available in advance could make the difference between an individual engaging or withdrawing from services.

DOI: 10.4324/9781003269724-16

In order to create information that is accessible and inclusive consider,

- The overall content and message.
- The format, size, colour, font, spacing.
- Length of written phrases in addition.
- Being clear, concise and consistent.

Some information will be appropriate to include as isolated topics within a 'process' or step-by-step document as standalone but linked pieces of information, e.g. accessing hardware through to how to complete a digital feedback form. It can be helpful to think about how many different topics are included and if they could be misinterpreted or need further explanation independently. In which case, consider if it may be of benefit to have the information on a separate document. Ultimately service users will be able to engage more successfully if they have three really accessible documents rather than wading through one that overwhelms and confuses.

The core elements in preparing the service user in order to participate include,

1. Consenting to and understanding participation in telehealth or video consultations.
2. Awareness of required hardware and software.
3. Assessment equipment (e.g. for swallow assessments).
4. Resources already sent by the clinician.
5. Ability to access e-forms/ratings scales to support clinician's assessment.
6. A third person to support assessment for risk mitigation (see also Chapter 16).

CONSENT

Just as we would consent a person for any other intervention, consent to participate and an understanding of what the telehealth/video consultation process involves is imperative. Throughout the recent pandemic, assumed or implicit consent has taken precedence, i.e. if it does not state explicitly in a service user's record that they *do not* wish to participate in telehealth/video consultations, it can be assumed that they will engage.

However, some clinicians, services or organisations prefer to have it actually documented so there is no margin of error and a service user is fully aware of what they are agreeing to. Collating consent may be in a number of different formats. This may be verbal but documented in the service user's record, completing of a paper form scanned in and attached or an e-consent form. E-consents can also take one of two forms, a true e-consent, where the service uses specialist software to send out a form electronically by email that is signed using touch screen ability, or by creating an electronic version that uses tick boxes to consent and can be uploaded as a PDF into the service user's electronic record.

This consent can act as consent for *all* services offering video consultations so that a service user only has to complete it once. The exception to this would be if the service had specific caveats or idiosyncrasies requiring a standalone consent for an individual service. This might be where a service user is taking part in a group session for example and they are consenting to sharing their information with multiple group members, not just a clinician.

One vital element of consent is checking that a service user has access to the necessary hardware.

HARDWARE AND SOFTWARE

Checking if a service user has the appropriate hardware to engage in a video consultation or telehealth session seems rather obvious, but it can be surprising how many service users will advise they didn't know they needed a computer or a smart phone when they are unable to join a call. Eliminating all potential queries as early on in the process as possible is far more beneficial for everyone.

Do they have access to,

- A smart phone.
- An android or Apple tablet are perhaps the most common but Google, Windows and other devices may also be what an individual has available.
- A desktop or laptop computer.
- A working microphone and webcam. These can be tested as part of the initial set up with many of the platforms having integral camera and microphone checks or recognition built in.
- Reliable access to broadband/mobile internet.

As well as,

- A quiet and confidential space to use their device.
- Somewhere to rest the device and somewhere comfortable to sit.
- Adequate lighting for their head and neck to be supported if needed and viewed clearly.

Erring on the side of caution and working on the basis that the service user's awareness is limited will ensure nothing integral to the session is left to chance and omitted. Checking at the earliest opportunity what a service user has access to will allow for more efficient clinical preparation, such as knowing if a service user's engagement will be via a smart phone-size screen or a larger device. It won't impact on the consultation taking place, but it might make a difference to the session content such as what the clinician chooses to share remotely if the screen size is limiting for visual comfort of the service user, such as forms, images or online timers.

For some platforms, additional download of software(s) to enhance the user experience can be beneficial. This is more likely to be where there is an app to complement the process or an app is being used for the actual video consultation.

- A quick guide with the link or QR code to download may be the quickest and easiest method.

- Whilst for web-based applications, bookmarking for ease of finding for repeat consultations is an option.

You may want to consider clarifying that it is the service user's responsibility to ensure their device is in good working order and it remains the service user's responsibility to ensure they have access to the internet. For most service users, these will be unquestioned elements but it can be helpful to make them a core requirement so there is no discrepancy or misinterpretation of a service's vs a service user's therapeutic obligations.

ASSESSMENT EQUIPMENT

Service users vary as much in what therapy interventions are as they do in demographic or cohort. Preparing service users to have physical objects to hand is as much a factor as checking they have reliable internet. The equipment will differ dependent on the aims of a session, such as if it is a communication or swallow assessment, or a group intervention that is the main premise. We have all undertaken sessions in person that have started out as one type and finished as an entirely different type, and video consultations are no exception.

The types of additional assessment equipment it may be useful having to hand are,

Dysphagia (swallow) Assessments (see referral infographic PDF and link for RCSLT Clinical Decision-Making Tool in online resources).

- Torches for further view of oral cavity.
- Plate, spoon, fork and knife.
- Cup or beaker, ideally opaque to allow for fluid to be seen.
- Teaspoon.
- Small hand mirror or compact mirror.
- Thickener (service user's own or sachets from prep kit that clinician sends).
- Range of food items to cover levels four–seven of the IDDSI descriptors.

COMMUNICATION ASSESSMENTS

For *communication assessments,* it may be useful to have electronic versions/screen-shareable PDFs of the documents below.

- Voice/dysfluency diary.
- Lax vox/air pressure exercise equipment (sports cup with lid and wide straw/tubing).
- Reading passages.

(Editable initial communication assessment in online resources.)

RESOURCES SENT AHEAD

Being prepared in some instances may also mean controlling some factors to limit risk by ensuring information is sent ahead. Where previously an automated response to post resources might have been the 'go to', there is now much more opportunity to consider sending PDFs and or URLs that can be accessed electronically and saved for reference or printed by the service user. This ensures that, wherever possible, services remain paperless or paperlite, maximising efficiency and cost savings whilst still providing effective and relevant information to enhance interventions. There are of course instances where posting physical items may be necessary such as thickener sachets or straws/tubing.

A QUICK SET UP KIT

This could either be an electronic file or physical kit that includes,

- User guides for how to join a call.
- Information guides for troubleshooting and risk mitigation (Chapters 14 and 16 – Using a Third Party).
- Thickener sachets if a swallow assessment is planned should be sent by post if the service user doesn't have currently prescribed thickener that is accessible.
- Tubing for air pressure exercises (alternatively, service users could be signposted to images of a suitable cup with wide straw-image).

BRINGING INDIVIDUALS ON A DIGITAL JOURNEY: CO-DESIGNING THEIR CARE

Digital isn't a destination, it's a journey! It is about learning what we as clinicians and users of healthcare services can access and use in order to better support and facilitate healthcare, be that our own or those on our caseload.

We may be more familiar with each passing month with electronic forms, completing things pre-appointment via opening a link that will return it by clicking 'submit' when we have finished inputting details but, perhaps not everyone is as far in their electronic enlightenment. It may be that they have yet to need to complete a form remotely, update their information or request an appointment is changed.

ELECTRONIC FORMS OR SELF-RATING SCALES

In-person initial sessions often see a clinician and a service user wading not only through a full history but also additional questions and subjective scales to further inform background, self-perception of the difficulty, impact on social and emotional interaction and goals.

Using electronic forms can not only reduce this element, allow service users an opportunity to complete independently without the pressure of a clinician watching but it also supports their digital journey. The impact being they can contribute to their therapy through highlighting aims and objectives, suggesting goals and providing valuable insight into where they are currently with regard to digital health engagement. The benefits are twofold. Not only does it allow for any documents

DOI: 10.4324/9781003269724-17

to be sent to the service user in advance and completed ahead of the session with the responses returned back to the clinician and saved in the service user's electronic record, it enables you as a clinician to acknowledge and refer to the content during the session, agree a baseline and set goals from the service user's own responses and have an understanding on digital ability with which to tailor the service user's continued digital journey.

COMPLETION

There are multiple ways of completing forms/questions including using online survey hosts such as Survey Monkey to return the information, MS Forms and multiple other electronic form creators are available such as Jot Form with several others readily found by searching the web. Typically there are set templates available for free within these sites, with premium options being available for a subscription.

Some organisations may have a patient portal that allows individuals to engage with healthcare providers in their locality to support managing appointments, medications and monitoring conditions. This may include primary care, mental health support, engaged community and acute secondary care services. It is also possible that an electronic form to gather pre- and post-appointment information can be completed through a service user portal/app via a URL and, as with other methods, returned to a central inbox for clinicians to review by PDF and then attach this information to a person's record for reference. This should be in line with local information governance for service user data collection and storage.

Independent practitioner appointments will not be able to interact with NHS service user portals unless affiliated or endorsed by NHS services, or the portal allows for ad hoc input from the service user to input any additional healthcare appointments, e.g. reports shared by a private consultant or therapist the service user may share.

In both instances, if electronic forms are not an established process, a standard editable document (e.g. MS Office Word) or as a PDF for printing can be used. It can then be sent to the service user, either via email or via SMS document attachment to be completed and returned in the same way it was sent if SMS is enabled for bidirectional communication. A service user would either complete the form electronically and save a copy to attach if in MSWord, or manually by printing off and filling in and then scanning or simply taking a photograph on their Smartphone or tablet device to attach via an email or SMS to return.

In all events of sharing information between clinicians/ service and service user, it is good practice to acknowledge the service has received the person's information.

It serves to increase reassurance for the service user that clinicians are not only acting on the information shared but appropriately documenting and storing it. Following receipt of emails, after attaching the document and copying any email content into the electronic record that is relevant to the person's care, ensure the email is deleted completely from the inbox to mitigate any risk of the information being forwarded or seen by anyone else. Whilst this guidance is based on NHS practice, most processes are good practice and will translate to independent practitioners, those working in education and other settings where care and therapy are being delivered. To ensure you are fully compliant, please confirm any new or changed processes with local information governance within your organisation.

THIRD PARTY SUPPORT

It may be relevant or necessary in certain situations to have a third party present with your service user during the virtual session. This may be for multiple reasons. One of the most prevalent for speech and language therapists are Clinical Swallowing Evaluations or Dysphagia Assessments. The practice of such assessments prior to the worldwide Covid-19 outbreak, which brought the UK into the first period of lockdown in March 2020, led to an increase in need for remote consultations to take place. In July 2020 the NHS announced a 'remote by default' approach to limit exposure and transmission of the virus.

However there was significant concern around how an assessment of swallow which has been associated in the UK by many NHS practitioners as requiring an in-person interaction, due to a myriad of risks and querying how an assessment could be safely undertaken by clinicians who had previously only ever assessed face to face.

Much research- and evidence-based practice has gone into developing proven ways of facilitating swallow assessments and there are increasing case studies and evaluations including Burns and Ward et al. (2019) and Bidmead, Reid, Marshall and Southern (2015) to support why remote assessments not only target real-time assessment and management, but can prevent escalation of swallowing difficulties and reduce admissions. A need to support healthcare staff was identified by RCSLT Fellow and senior research lecturer Dr Liz Boaden alongside SLT and Digital Health Clinical Lead Veronica Southern developing Teleswallowing training which has been deployed in multiple settings, both the NHS and private settings, and the focus of several case studies. In addition, HEE have devised and developed a programme to support training in practice with multiple partners across health and the dysphagia management sector, both training programmes are available as e-learning packages mapped to the Eating, Drinking and Swallowing Competencies Framework developed by RCSLT (see resources for links to both). RCSLT have also been at the forefront of developing guidance for remote swallow assessments alongside a clinical decision-making tool to support both clinician and third party facilitator in assessing appropriacy as well as preparing and performing the assessment process.

15

PREPARE TO PREPARE

IT MIGHT SEEM OBVIOUS, BUT HAVING EVERYTHING TO HAND IS THE KEY.

We may not be telepathic telepractitioners but we do know that sessions very often don't go as planned, so planning disaster mitigation strategies (new activities, exercises, etc.) is a useful tool to deploy in virtual consultations!

Once you have prepped the person and the appointment is confirmed, make sure you are ready. By ready, this isn't just being on time, switching the computer on and pressing join. This is the preparation and having everything to hand. Take an assessment: do you ever get the feeling during one that you think you know where all the bits and pieces you'll need are (you just need to sift through the filing cabinet or those piles of paper that you don't quite know the full contents of)? You might have forgotten something from the drawer in the other room or suddenly realise that exercise or activity you thought might be useful but decided not to pull out the advice sheet for, is now exactly the one you needed?

We have all been there, in a clinic room, and had to excuse ourselves, leaving the service user with or without additional family or friends to entertain themselves with the posters on the wall, as we discreetly popped out to retrieve Fred the Head, to give an impromptu swallow demonstration, fetch a game of pop up pirate to do discrimination tasks or freed an additional assessment from the wardrobe of resources that you risk disappearing into Narnia-style. How familiar is that scenario in some guise or other?

In a video consultation session, this isn't practical or professional, not to mention efficient. We need to be really prepared for almost every eventuality, that just in case sort of preparation in the event the course of the session takes a turn down an alternative path or, the service user struggles with the exercise you planned and you need to pull another 'out of the bag'.

Preparing to prepare is about,

- Having the right resources for the right individual and preparing what you can in advance to help you feel more in control and calm.
- Being efficient, try using resources more than once during a block of sessions where possible.
- What screens do you need to share? you will usually need to select/have open the screens to be shared in advance.
- Anything with sound to be played may need to 'select play with sound' – do this step before you share the screen!

Remember don't panic. If something goes wrong only you know and if you need to change activity finish the question or turn you are on and swap games/activities.

> TOP TIP: Remember this will be whatever you have open on your desktop, unless you are using MS Teams as this will give you options for all tabs you have open and allow you to select from multiple thumbnails. In MS Teams, to change screens you will need to stop sharing, select another and start sharing again. Other platforms may allow you to move between tabs as you share but you need to ensure that you are only sharing what is intended and not accidentally sharing a screen that you've been looking at in your lunch break! You also need to be mindful that you have closed any electronic records that are *not* relevant to the service user you are due to enter a virtual consultation with. Accidentally sharing information, however brief, would be a serious breach of person confidentiality, which you as the clinician would be responsible for and potentially be open to an investigation should this occur. The easiest thing to do is simply close any irrelevant tabs before activating the link. Furthermore, it will actually

enhance your connection, as the less you have open or running in the background, the less the internet connection has to contend with. For all platforms, pre-select your screens and have them accessible under new tabs you can easily select when you need to share.

So what do you actually need in your session? Let's break it down, not all of it will be relevant to every session or you might end up not needing to use something, but it makes it much easier to *be aware and prepare*!

WHAT WILL YOU SHARE?

a) Assessments – information for digital assessments, pre-adapted versions and how to translate existing assessments into formats suitable for use in video session will be given in resources.
b) Buzzers, bells, timers – there are a number of online resources for interactive buzzers, bells, clocks and timers that can be used in the same way as during in-person sessions. They are useful for multiple purposes, including monitoring breathing, setting session time limits and playing games.
c) Online games or activities – as above, there are numerous sites that, with a quick search of 'online speech therapy games', uncover a host of activities that might be useful to include in your session, replacing the games often utilised to support a myriad of language skills across all age groups. When you have identified the game/games you want to use in the session, just ensure they are open on separate tabs so you can screen share them as easily as possible and you aren't having to start searching for them mid-session. Of course there will be the times when a search is needed as you are making a dynamic assessment and a suggestion will occur to you, but only you need to know you weren't ready and raring to go with a particular activity as whoever is on the other side of your screen can only see what you share!

d) Whiteboard – these can be super useful tools to have for all sorts of exercises, whether they are speech- or language-based. There may be one included in the platform, e.g. MS Teams.

TOP TIP: You need to have more than three people on a call usually to use a whiteboard so I use OneNote instead, screen share, and give remote control and this has a similar outcome!

You can also search for an online collaboration tool if you want more flexibility or are running group consultations and want everyone to be able to contribute at the same time, there are some great ones such as Google Jamboard, Miroboard or by using a template in Canva. Just set the board up and share the link with the service user's using the chat function (or even before the session if it is set up long enough in advance). This tool relies on a greater degree of technical ability and may not be appropriate for all service users but where it does work well it's great and very versatile.

e) Files – examples of these may be exercises, activities, diary sheets, resources such as diagrams to use or signpost to.

There may be other examples you can add to this list of suggestions so don't be limited, use your clinical creativity to enhance session content just as in person!

16

LIGHTS, CAMERA, ACTION … SMILE!

THE ENVIRONMENT

Would you do an in-person session in a poorly lit room with people wandering around the room? The simple answer is of course you wouldn't. So why would we consider doing anything even remotely different from an in-person appointment for a video appointment? The whole purpose is to replicate the process of an in-person session in digital form, so this means having a quiet, confidential space to do this.

Not just so you can focus and hear what is happening but for security and information governance purposes, too. You are engaging in a clinical session so all the same considerations should be made with the same processes adhered to, in order for the session to be deemed clinically safe and secure.

A space that is considered confidential could be a clinic room specifically for video consultations, an office that has been booked for the purpose of a video consultation, an MDT room with multiple professions expected to join the call, or even the living room or spare room in your own house, separated by a door from the rest of the household. All of them are equally suitable as long as you and the service user have got no interruptions and no one is able to walk in or overhear.

DOI: 10.4324/9781003269724-19

LIGHTING

It sounds trivial to be considering how well you are lit up but it serves a really crucial purpose, as if you or your service user is poorly lit, the session may be less successful due to reduced clarity of vision for either party. This is not only for communicative success but also for safety, particularly where for some clinicians' assessments of swallow may be conducted. It may be the difference between seeing how to safely copy therapy exercises or accurately assess jaw opening or laryngeal elevation, so if neither can see the other clearly, the impact could be more than just if the picture is a little dark.

There are a whole manner of tips and tricks for being in the best light during a virtual consultation; let's face it, YouTubers have been mastering it for years, and from halo lights to clip-on mini versions for better selfies, it is the simplest of tools that is your best friend, natural light!

TOP TIP: Light yourself from the front using natural daylight where possible. Positioning yourself in front of a window is an easy way to do this but if this is not possible, try and position your equipment with the main ceiling light in front of you. Having it in the background can cause strange screen disturbances such as halos of light, glare or reflections that distort how you are seen by the service user or others on the call. It can be distracting as well as making it more difficult to see your face and mouth clearly, which are important elements, especially when we are in a virtual setting. If you are working from home or are able to request lighting options, daylight bulbs can work well as a substitute or even selfie lights! These are readily available from many online retailers and usually clip to a screen or nearby rest to illuminate you from the front. The same is true for service users and how to advise and prepare their environment and equipment is addressed in Chapter 13.

TOP TIP: Facing a window and having the light in front of you rather than behind ensures that you are lit from the front and gives a similar effect to using artificial light in that not only does it give the best viewing light for those on the other side of the screen, but, it's also a little more complimentary as harsh shadows are less likely to cast across your face as they might with artificial lighting or lighting from behind.

It enables the person to see your face as clearly as possible and means that they can use facial and visual cues much more readily, including lip reading, than if you are partially in a shadow or under/over lit due to poor lighting.

This would be advisable for those you are engaging with too as it will provide similar benefits for you as a clinician being able to see them as clearly as possible and enhance clinical observations. It is particularly important for individuals you might be needing to assess for oral motor skills and movement and or as part of swallowing assessments. Using pen torches or smartphone torches can be really useful in these instances for getting clear, well-lit imagery of oral cavities either by the person directly or with the support of a third party (relative, carer, support worker etc.).

VISUAL HYGIENE AND VISUAL NOISE

As odd as these phrases sound, they are a phenomenon and can really affect engagement virtually. Visual hygiene and noise isn't about how clean your spectacles are, although in all seriousness it really does help to make sure,

- You can see the screen well enough.
- Where possible have glasses that are coated to reduce glare, especially if you are a screen user for a large amount of your time and to enhance the view for the individuals on the other side of the screen.

Being 'visually clean' is how your environment is seen on screen and the steps required to ensure your environment can enhance or negatively impact on your virtual session. There are some inbuilt tools within some platforms that allow you to blur the background or change it for something else.

Did you know that blur background features weren't designed as a clever way to hide the washing pile in the background but were actually a communication aid? The feature was originally developed to enhance the experience of a member of staff at Microsoft with a hearing impairment to minimise external visual noise from virtual meetings for those who are auditorily impaired and lip read.

This simple modification to online engagement is now used by people globally and is a highly useful tool for virtual clinical consultations, and, in addition to functioning as an accessibility tool, it also supports confidentiality and security for you as a clinician. How?

Imagine you are working from home and seeing a service user for the first time. You do not blur the background or use background image. You are aware from the demographics that the service user lives geographically close to you. They may have children at the same school or childcare provision or work in a care home that your mum, dad or grandparents are resident at, but they do not know this and you want to keep your work very separate from your clinical work. You have your first consultation and in the background is the wall of family photos! The service user has been able to have a good look and now knows all your children's or relatives' faces, what your family home looks like and begins to discuss events that are outside of the clinical appointment premise, but you feel uncomfortable asking them to not discuss this as you feel it may break down your therapy relationship.

This could be avoided by ensuring the environment is as much of a blank canvas as possible. It will not only keep your personal environment secure and protect confidentiality, but also be less of a distraction for the service user. This can be particularly effective for enhancing a service user's clear view and tuning into what you are saying, as well as reducing visual stimulus for service users that this may impact, such as those on the Autism spectrum as busy, 'noisy' backgrounds can be very distracting and act as a sensory overload. More suggestions and information about supporting neurodiverse individuals can be found in Section 3, Chapter 36: You, Me and ASD.

The next steps are the awareness that safety and security are integral to delivering care remotely and knowing your IG leads can be key!

17

To IG or to Not IG, THAT Is the Question

It's easy to assume that everyone knows what information governance (IG) is. Everyone that works in the NHS has to be IG compliant as part of their mandatory skills training, but do we actually know what we are addressing in this context? NHSE (now part of the NHS England and NHS Improvement Transformation Directorate) succinctly defines IG as being the process that supports how we *'manage and share information appropriately'*. If only it were that simple! Life in the digital realm would be a lot more straightforward, but it wouldn't be half as much fun or brain busting. So what is it we really want to know when we ask, 'To IG or not to IG? There are a few questions to answer to ensure we are keeping information as safe as possible and in turn keep the person to whom that information belongs to safe.

Having worked closely with the Data Protection Officer (DPO) or *'DP O No'*, as I affectionately termed the lead at an organisation I was at. I learned it was much easier to work on a 'no go' policy for data security. Initially investigate the clinical task thoroughly prior to putting a plan in place rather than the alternative of the 'whatever works' methodology that was suggested at the outset of Covid-19 to manage clinical flow and engagement. Opening the floodgate early, having bypassed potentially vital considerations that on the surface might seem innocuous and innocent but in reality could have led to sharing data with a whole region or beyond and was the main reason a proceed caution sign was hung on my back! Yes, it is attached to the concern that caution brings delays and there are others that walk the opposite path in response to IG but

DOI: 10.4324/9781003269724-20

something that I was advised stuck with me: if I always consider every episode of information sharing as if it was my own information that was being shared, I will always strive for the same level of security and integrity to be applied regardless of source or purpose.

The main questions that I ask so I can understand the process and support an appropriate policy are,

- What information?
- From and to where?
- About who, and with who, are we sharing information?
- For what purpose?

These questions are all significant but can be summarised in the questions below for information governance purposes which then help advise,

- How will it be shared?
- Where will it be shared?
- Where is it stored and for how long?

If you are in any doubt about cybersecurity, data and information governance relating to patient information, in the first instance please contact your local information governance lead who will be able to advise further.

For security breaches related specifically to anything related to video consultations please follow your organisations standard operating procedure and escalate as appropriate.

DON'T BE IG-NORANT

You know the questions you are going to ask, but what are you going to do with the answers?

For this chapter, the focus will be on the three considerations below. I can't answer all of these as some will be reliant on your organisational policies, but if you are equipped to ask the right questions you can protect yourself and the people you are providing care for in your service.

- **How will it be shared** – think about if you are sending emails, text messages, letters via digital means (i.e. are they attached to an email but have PID or person identifiable information?).
- **Where will it be shared** – does your organisation have an electronic healthcare record (EPR) or a person administration system (PAS), is there a patient portal where people can access their own care records from, is the organisation linked to a wider shared healthcare record that multiple organisations access (primary and secondary care, mental health, ambulance service, etc.)?
- **Where is it stored, who has access and for how long is it stored?** Is your organisation storing information on servers, using cloud-based storage or other means, e.g. paper-based methods? What are the policies for keeping this data? Is there a finite timescale as with paper copies or forever if digital records?

One activity I would highly recommend you undertake is to determine whether the process has a Data Privacy Impact Assessment (DPIA) in place or if one is considered to be

DOI: 10.4324/9781003269724-21

required. Where virtual-video consultations are concerned, the answer is almost 100% yes!

DPI-AY?

What is one, who writes it, where does it need to be shared and how often does it need updating?

DPIAs have fairly standard formats and the likelihood is that your organisation will have their own template for you to input the relevant data into. The first time you complete one they can be a bit daunting, but remember they are there to safeguard your service user and your organisation.

- Complete the information that you do know.
- Clarify any wording.
- Establish any missing information.
- Identify acronyms.
- Define processes i.e. what information is it asking for, is there a standard operating procedure (SOP) that the DPIA supports?

Remember, you are not on your own. If you need support, it's absolutely worth a quick email to arrange a telephone or video call with your IG lead or Data Protection Officer (DPO), whether NHS, public or third party sector, most organisations will have a lead and usually they will be more than happy to support. They would much rather you ask questions than compromise and risk a data breach, plus it's a good way to build collaborative networks for future digital projects. From experience, people that work in IG and data are time-generous and love to share their knowledge with others. Their work is so integral to digital projects and typically they are a very small team in comparison to the scale of work they do, with individuals often overlooked, so it can be a rare opportunity to not only gain an insight but also shine a light on their work and highlight their vital work in contributing to person and staff safety.

You can find templates and example video consultation DPIAs in the online resources section.

DCB, EASY AS 123: CLINICAL SAFETY STANDARDS

Do you know your CSO from your DPO? We touched on the Data Protection Officer role in Chapters 17 and 18, but now there's a new kid on the digital block, the Clinical Safety Officer (CSO). Their role is to mitigate risk and set apart the risks posed by implementing new digital technologies and/or processes and develop a hazard log of these as a live document during pilot and beyond.

Whether you are the manufacturer of a virtual consultation platform or healthcare organisation, a Clinical Safety Officer (CSO) must be a named clinician with current registration with a professional body. They must also be trained in clinical risk management which can be provided by NHS Digital or a number of independent providers (see the online resources section for more information on training). It is worth familiarising yourself with who the CSO's in your organisation are as they will need to undertake a hazard workshop for all new digital projects or technologies, so if the platform you are using for virtual consultations is new then this is an opportunity to get involved with the process. The purpose is,

- To highlight anything that could go wrong with the technology.
- What the outcome would be.
- What the risk would be to the service/service user.
- Likelihood of it recurring.
- Mitigate risk in advance.

DOI: 10.4324/9781003269724-22

The CSO will be responsible for overseeing the clinical risk management activities and signing off the documentation. They will typically run clinical risk management workshops to formulate the hazard register and validate the evidence set out in the safety case. The CSO is responsible for ensuring that the work is carried out, but they are not personally accountable for any clinical risk, this should be collective.

The main purpose of the CSO is to coordinate the two digital clinical safety standards set out by NHS Digital. The new Digital Clinical Safety Strategy produced by NHSE/I Transformation Directorate (formerly known as NHSX) also highlights the significance of clinical safety and why it's more than just seeking to apportion blame but about ensuring we learn from any situations where potential or actual harm is the outcome. These safety standards are separated into manufacturer and organisation DCB0129 and DCB0160. The requirements in the two standards are almost identical.

Each standard has over 60 requirements but, following identifying the CSO, you must

- Gather information and document the processes.
- Assess risk and produce a hazard log.
- Clinical risk management in live service.
- Post-deployment assurance check.

TOP TIP: It's tempting to think, 'it can't be that bad, we'll do it later'. Attempting to write a hazard log after the technology has been implemented will be inaccurate as you will miss things out which could mean they aren't accounted for and could happen again. An effective and safe clinical risk management process can't be done on the fly, ad hoc or in retrospect. It needs to be methodical, rigorous, systematic and above all replicable, so you can repeat it with relative straightforward ease over and over again as the process is tested and reiterated.

NHSE/I Transformation Directorate (formerly NHSX) are working to support clinicians working in digital patient safety within the NHS to increase awareness and support the development of the training available so that more clinicians can train as CSOs and support digital transformations.

If you have an NHS.net email and registered with the NHS e-learning health platform you can register for the online and foundation workshops (these will need organisational approval and funding; cost at time of writing for foundation workshops are £475 per NHS delegate and £625 for Commercial/External.).

For more information about digital patient safety and the role of CSOs there is information available from NHS Digital, NHSE/I Transformation Directorate (formerly NHSX) and independent organisations specialising in clinical safety. Please see online resources for links to websites.

20

ASSESSING AND MITIGATING RISK

So how is digital clinical risk assessed and can we mitigate against it? Let's take it as one question with two parts. The first part is straightforward in many respects. As clinicians, we assess clinical risk *all* the time and are constantly making judgements as to how to proceed with situations based on what is safe and appropriate at the time for that person. So, adding digital into the mix is really just adding additional layers to the safety cake. We already assess risk dynamically but digital clinical risk management just needs a little more consideration. As outlined in Chapter 19, it has to be a structured and systematic process to ensure that any hazards that are encountered are lessons learned and mitigated against for future episodes (Figure 20.1).

The Clinical Safety Cake

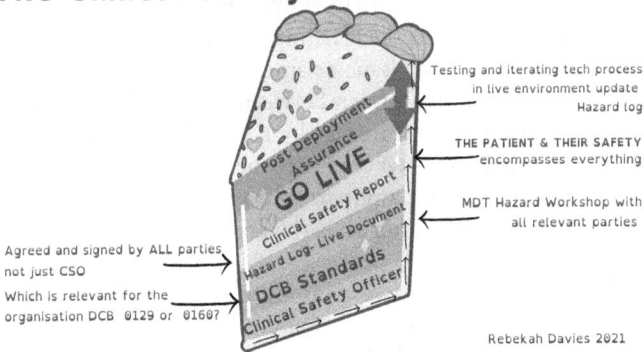

Testing and iterating tech process in live environment update Hazard log

THE PATIENT & THEIR SAFETY encompasses everything

MDT Hazard Workshop with all relevant parties

Agreed and signed by ALL parties not just CSO

Which is relevant for the organisation DCB 0129 or 0160?

Rebekah Davies 2021

Figure 20.1 Clinical Safety Cake (R Davies 2021)

Digital patient safety is a piece of cake when you make a safety case into a safety cake! Clinical safety can all too often be an afterthought because of the lack of awareness and training around this key factor of patient care. It isn't something we can pick and choose to include in our digital deployments, patient safety is core to every other clinical area and there is no difference with digital safety. It should be baked in, not sprinkled on, in order to maximise safety and efficiency in every aspect of digital practice.

THE BLAME GAME

When things go wrong there is the temptation to apportion blame to someone whom this could sit neatly at the feet of, it could be the person that knows the most or the least or attached to a particular part of the process. If the platform you are using for your virtual clinics crashes and a person can't log into it for their appointment, is this the technology that is at fault or the IT team that is responsible? If the link didn't get sent out because the system went down but this wasn't realised until the person should have joined, is that the responsibility of the administrator or clinician? In reality it should be a collaborative process where everyone should be an accountable and responsible part of the process, find solutions and mitigate for future instances. Rather than simply looking to blame someone or something, find the learning objective and use it to mitigate against the same issue arising on subsequent occasions. A comparison is often drawn between the aerospace industry where a 'no blame' culture has long been fostered. It ensures a fair and safe process where everyone is comfortable in sharing information about any part of a project so clinical safety and mitigation of future risk is the objective, not pointing the finger of blame.

Digital clinical safety/digital clinical risk management is closely linked to the processes associated with IG, including the DPIA, but the really important distinction that has been little known about and little utilised because of limited awareness of the role existing is the hazard workshops and the value of these.

The workshops serve multiple roles,

- Bring everyone involved in the project together (clinically and non-clinically).
- Clarify roles and senior responsibilities for the wider project (SRO, etc.).
- Outlines the project, including specifics of any time-critical factors, for those that need clarification.
- Provides an opportunity to highlight any possible factors that could impact clinical safety.
- The hazard log is a live document so can be updated when any iterations are made.

DON'T PANIC

- Digital clinical safety is there for exactly that reason, to ensure safety across clinical situations when using digital technologies, pathways or tools to enhance and deliver healthcare.
- You will *never* have to undertake a hazard log or clinical safety report and safety case alone, there will always be a CSO to advise and guide as part of the process and they should be signed off by a qualified CSO and the Chief Clinical Information Officer (CCIO) or senior digital clinical leader, e.g. Chief Nursing Information Officer (CNIO) or Chief/Allied Health Profession Information Officer (CAHPIO).
- If you are inspired by the 'Clinical Safety Cake' model and think digital safety could be a *piece of cake*, please see the resources section for links to follow for further information about digital clinical safety.

21

SAFE AND SOUND:
SAFEGUARDING AND CONSENT

In reference to booking, consent will be highlighted but covered in more depth within information governance, GDPR and security. Consent may be collated in numerous ways, and for numerous purposes and it is this that you should be clear about initially. Ask,

'*WHO* WILL I BE CONSENTING FOR A VIRTUAL SESSION?'

Is this the service user themselves, a lasting power of attorney, a care home assuming responsibility on behalf of numerous persons, a parent or guardian or someone else?

'*WHAT* AM I CONSENTING FOR?'

Have a clear objective as to what purpose you are seeking consent, is it pre-consent to acknowledge an individual can undertake virtual consultations, is it permission to share outcomes with students or peers for training purposes or, are you seeking consent to share their image or quotes they have shared in their feedback?

'*WHY* AM I CONSENTING?

Are you seeking permission to record a session? Be clear of these objectives, for whose benefit is this and who will have access to it? (See platforms and IG sections around using MS Teams/MS N365 DPIA.)

DOI: 10.4324/9781003269724-24

'*WHEN* WILL I BE COLLECTING CONSENT?'

At the outset of the Covid-19 pandemic, consenting regulations relaxed in line with information governance and security, with NHSE/I Transformation Directorate (formerly NHSX) promoting a 'whatever works' and 'assumed consent' model of working remotely. However, it wasn't long until IG departments and clinical safety officers found escalating concerns with this way of approaching, with numerous incidents of security being breached using some platforms, leading to a need to have boundaries in place where these were felt to have fallen by the wayside. So when should you collect consent? As soon as possible! It should also be recapped regularly in case the service user has changed their preferences in anyway e.g. perhaps they previously didn't consent to emails but now want to.

'HOW AM I RECORDING THE CONSENT?'

Consent was one of these boundaries, with 'implicit' or 'assumed' being the most prevalent method of documenting consent. But not everyone understands the significance of this and why it could have consequences if it wasn't documented accurately and appropriately. Implicit relies on taking it as assumed that it is OK to undertake a virtual consultation in the absence of a definitive or categorical yes or no response. It is still an accepted form of consenting an individual, but it is wise to be cautious and instead opt for more explicit one-off consent that is then valid for all subsequent consultations and can be used as a baseline for clarity, accuracy and security at the outset of a session. Remeber to check in regularly to make sure what was originally consented for is still relevant. If any changes need making document in electronic notes where available or other clinical systems. You can also record dates checked for changes if there are none. Check if consenting for video consultations in one service covers other services in your organisation too as any changes will affect these!

22

DURING A REMOTE CONSULTATION: THE CLINICIAN WILL SEE YOU NOW!

The advice and tips from Chapter 16: Lights, Camera, Action … Smile! highlight a number of suggestions around utilising natural light to enhance your video consultations and make the best use of resources available. The environment, as we have already learned, is key to the success and security of the session, but lighting alone can't take responsibility or credit for these outcomes.

Seating and positioning are also crucial factors. Just as with in-person appointments, you wouldn't assess a person if they were slumped in bed or folded like origami in a chair, it's important to recognise how and where a person sits during an assessment, particularly assisted physical and/or swallow assessments vs language-based assessments.

Using similar principles to get the best positioning such as,

* Getting as close to the midline as possible.
* Sitting as upright as possible.
* In a chair sitting squarely with feet to floor if possible.
* In bed upright and in the midline, well positioned with pillows to support head and limbs where appropriate for both comfort and to aid maintaining a good postural position.

Don't forget you are in charge and, if after trying to find ways of getting a person into a better posture to safely assess or ensuring the lighting is adequate, you can confidently see all the main oral structures and observe stages of swallow, you can stop the assessment going any further and rearrange.

 DOI: 10.4324/9781003269724-25

It is far better to be safe and be cautious than to risk any additional factors that could negatively impact on an individual whilst you are managing the events.

You can make recommendations based on what you have seen and what you feel is clinically safe and follow up with further sessions as soon as possible. It may be that the person isn't as well as they have been and are taking medication, making them less reactive than usual, meaning they are struggling to support themselves to sit as well as usual but may be more able to manage in a few days when they have completed the course. It may be a long-term medication change and needs to factored in to further sessions, such as having the person positioned prior to the session so that if they can only manage for a short time in the assessment, this is maximised because the session has been prepared for (see content in Chapters 16 and 17 around reducing risk and third party support).

Prior session information about preparing will likely have been shared but reiterating this and leaving persons and carers with clear guidelines for preparing for the next session by drawing their attention to the information they already have or offering to resend if they have forgotten will be useful.

WHAT IF IT GOES WRONG, TIPS FOR TROUBLESHOOTING

Just like an in-person session, things go wrong in video! It may be at the stage of logging on for either person or clinician, two persons may 'arrive' at once or it might be difficulties such as struggling to screen share to complete an assessment or share exercises.

Remember, it's not the end of the world, we are only human and it is accepted that we are allowed to make mistakes.

My fail safe is logging out and rejoining as you may have discovered yourself! This often resolves issues around being able to hear and see everyone effectively on both sides of the screen, but, if this doesn't work or if it's not the thing that has gone wrong, how can you troubleshoot or manage?

The best way to ensure you retain contact throughout a planned appointment is by having a contact number ready for the person so you can either ring them or send a new join-ing link. This is vital, as is ensuring that any information you send out has the contact number and email address for the ser-vice so the person has a way of contacting you to say they are struggling.

As the clinician, if it is factors out of your control such as Wi-Fi breaking up or even unplanned outages of a network, the best thing to do is admit digital defeat and revert either to a telephone call if the person is happy to do so or by rearranging. This latter option may be more appropriate if you were near-ing the end of a consultation and nearing the start of another, rather than initiating a phone call which may make you late for starting the next appointment on time.

If it is difficult using inbuilt elements of the platform, such as screen sharing, consider ways of sharing this information in other ways so that you can still achieve the outcome you need. This may be sending the document as an attachment, and if it is a form that requires completing, asking the per-son/carer/family to complete and return it within a set period. Alternatively, if it is an assessment that relies on completion of a form such as subjective voice quality questionnaires like the Voice Handicap Index, it could be a case of reading the ques-tions out verbally and recording the response for the person and inputting straight into the person's record.

Ultimately, you make the decisions as to how viable the session is to carry on, there are no hard and fast rules and we use our clinical judgement just as we do with in-person appointments.

It's a good idea to make a record of any issues you have encountered in previous attempts such as difficulties logging in or leaving a session; this may be about the browsers they are using or need prompting to close the session properly before the clinician leaves the session so you know they have gone and can't rejoin. Some platforms have built this with one-time links as a safety feature that, once the clinician has left or the session is shut down, no one can re-enter. This can be useful in group sessions where the chat function has been used so no one can access or add to it once the session is over. This is slightly different if you have used a standard MS Teams link and sent out as a recurring meeting to multiple people as the chat is visible after and may need managing in terms of putting additional rules in, such as only using the chat function during the sessions.

For many this wouldn't be a consideration but having evaluated multiple platforms for features, safety and IG it has raised scenarios that we might not previously have anticipated as a problem but resulted in cold sweats in a cupboard when they have occurred and needed addressing!

Many services don't yet have any support for clinicians to access for general technical queries other than NHS Trust IT departments or their own organisations. Similarly for individuals, there is little evidence at present to suggest that there are standard procedures or support methods within organisations for those receiving technical support outside of their clinical appointment. This can impact on individuals accessing appointments due to lack of digital literacy or through not having the appropriate equipment. How individuals can be better supported to access virtual appointments through enhancing digital literacy, supporting technical barriers and reviewing inequalities around equipment and infrastructure are being reviewed and developed nationally in the form of a targeted blueprint at the time of writing by NHS England and NHS Improvement. Solutions such as virtual receptionists and schedulers alongside hubs and loanservices for hardware are just some of the potential outcomes that may support these areas that may impact or lead to inequalities and exclusion.

BUTTONS, BUTTONS EVERYWHERE!

I remember one of my colleagues saying very worriedly, 'but there are buttons EVERYWHERE, how do I know which ones to use?', when the idea of navigating a keyboard, plus a video consulting platform plus the electronic health record was presented. That was before she was advised that a headset could be helpful, too. It worked like a super power, maybe giving her the feeling she was in control. Whatever it was it worked and there were still a lot of buttons but I think a few boost buttons helped too! Happily, she completely mastered the art of the possible with virtual therapy and contributed actively to pathway redesign of several offers within the service.

TOP THREE BUTTONS I USE MOST AND WHY!

1. Control + C or Control + V – by using Control and C to copy and Control and V to paste into browsers and chat functions quickly and easily, I can do things much quicker than just typing.
2. Tab – quickly move up and down or across.
3. Print screen – it's a great way to easily save something as an image, share something or add it into a document (I have other similar tips for moving, sharing and using images later!).
4. Control + down arrow – (yes, another pair) but another time-saving device for highlighting lists to copy and move quickly. This is great for copying a chat into someone's notes if the platform doesn't keep a complete record like some do (e.g. MS Teams, which is great for completeness of records).
5. Windows button – this unlocks a personalised experience for you as a user but can also support therapy interventions, increasing accessibility and inclusion, *wait and see more in Chapter 34.*

DOI: 10.4324/9781003269724-26

TOP TIP: Remember if you are using the chat function for any reason (it is a great accessibility tool) and it can be useful for session management such as adding links etc., remind the person/people you are 'chatting' with that anything in the chat section may be copied (obviously using Control +C) and kept in their healthcare record. This can particularly help manage group sessions and prevent any inappropriate discussion! I tend to pop a message in at the start 'Hi XXXXXX please use the chat to ask me any questions about today's session. Please ring 0XX XXXXXXX if for any reason there are any technical difficulties. Thanks Rebekah.'

24

'YOU'RE ON MUTE'

SILENT BUT NOT DEADLY

We all know 'you're on mute' has become the mantra of virtual working. It's almost considered a digital sin in some circles, you can hear the exasperation in some people's voices as they delight in informing you of the offence you have committed, to the extent that I challenge myself not to commit it, but still get frustrated and berate myself after if I do. It happens even to 'experts'; it's not the end of the world, we may be silent for few seconds but it isn't mute-iny!

DID YOU KNOW?

Being able to mute is actually an accessibility enhancer, particularly in group consultations or where there may be additional sound sources, even in a one-to-one that may be a distraction. This can be on both the clinician and the person engaging's part and be for a number of uses. Primarily, the obvious reason being is that mute cuts out background noise and feedback. So it makes it easier to attend to what is being said by one person if just the person's microphone who is talking is on in case there are sounds and distractions happening in the background of the other person/people. The other benefit is reduction of feedback. Typically this happens when a group of people are on a call, so can be useful to be aware of as part of group rules, but just being aware that strange noises can occur if microphones are very close to someone's mouth (especially if wearing a headset) can really reduce some of the squeals and squeaks that can interfere.

DOI: 10.4324/9781003269724-27

In addition to mute are specific noise reduction or natural voice options in some platforms. It's worth noting these aren't available in all platforms and may have different names depending on the platform. For example, Zoom has a function called 'Original Voice', with the premise of producing the most natural-sounding voice quality. Similarly, Microsoft Teams has a noise-reduction feature which eliminates external sounds to produce a voice quality as close to the person's natural one as possible. These are particularly useful functions for those of you who, if like me, specialise in voice as an area of practice. As a clinician in the NHS, I'm more familiar with Microsoft Teams, but where other platforms are implemented similar features may be available such as Google Meet, which can now filter out your dog barking or key strokes. If you haven't used these before and don't know if they will make a difference, don't be afraid to test them out and see if they enhance the delivery of your practice.

Recording will be different depending on the platform, there's more information coming up in Section 4 about recording and you can use the information guides in the resources for recording a personalised video if you have never done it before.

TOP TIP: You can have a test run with a willing colleague or family member and test the quality of the sound with and without the feature by recording the session and watching it back.

25

GUESS WHO? CLARIFYING IDENTITY

A significant onus is placed on person safety and one of the prevalent discussions is in relation to how we can effectively confirm a service user's identity.

Is it enough to have the 'service user' say, yes, I am Mr Smith?

In a face-to-face setting, we might expect the service users only to arrive at an appointment if when they arrive they present with some sort of evidence of the appointment information from the service and, conversely, the appropriate information was held for the service user by the service. However, even in this scenario there are still processes for qualifying a service user prior to engaging. This may be a physical receptionist checking service users in, or a self-check in screen which is increasingly used in healthcare settings to cross-reference the information held about service users. This information will either be from central NHS records shared with NHS organisations or from localised databases for private practice. In both instances clarity for who, with whom and what the appointment is for is essential. This will limit misunderstanding of the appointment purpose and mistaken identity of either service user or clinician.

So, how do we do this virtually ... get them to wave their appointment letter in front of the screen or flash the email? We could, but can we be sure that is the real letter? So, does this *really* validate they are who they say they are? For information governance and clinical safety purposes, the short answer is no. We need to take additional measures to clarify identity so we can be certain when documenting that we are discussing

DOI: 10.4324/9781003269724-28

and sharing information that is relevant and refers to this particular person. The easiest way to do this is, like with all digital pathways, to replicate what would happen in-person.

An administrator or self-check in service would validate the service user's responses against what is held in the person record. It is acknowledged that many organisations do have electronic records, but those who do not should instead have an electronic rostering system driven by national agenda and their respective professional body.

So, virtually we can replicate these processes in a number of ways. One method is using automated digital processes for this, a service user will follow the link for their consultation and be prompted to enter relevant demographic information such as,

- Full name
- DOB
- Email
- Mobile
- Postcode

This will allow what is entered to be mapped against data that is held, with the two sets of information matching in order for service users to gain access to the consult. An alternative is that, when in the consult, if pre-validation as part of the logging-in process has not been possible due to the platform being used (see also Chapter 8 for platform features), the clinician should clarify the details against what the record information indicates is accurate. It is advisable to check with local processes and governance policies in the event any changes to the record (telephone number, email, address) have occurred, as it may be necessary for the service user to ensure the information has been updated with their GP so that central records are accurate, as local amends will not typically update the NHS spine. Similarly, in private organisations please ensure the main database holds the most up-to-date demographic information to ensure incidences of service users' details being shared accidentally do not occur, for example if a person has moved house and letters and reports are still being sent to this address.

> TOP TIP: If you are doing manual checks of identity, so you are not giving any information out, ask that the service users to clarify information that only they would know, such as middle name, next of kin, confirm mobile number or even establish a password system prior to the session so that when they join the call before you continue, ask that they confirm the password sent via SMS/email.

In the future it is anticipated that AI will play an increasing part in security, for example face mapping or other biometrics may be a more standard process to validate who is attending alongside the demographic data to minimise further any data breaches or instances of misidentification, but Massey (2018) highlights that merely buying new AI tools 'does not improve defences, they need to be deployed, maintained and monitored' to be effective, and this is why the role of both clinical safety officers and information governance leads are so vital to ensure the technologies we deploy are clinically safe for individuals to engage with.

Wherever possible, try to think about how you can be confident the service user is the person you are supposed to be meeting with and ensure you have documented how you did this in the person's record. This will add to verification in subsequent sessions as well as being a record of events for any other professionals.

As strange as it might sound that someone should be impersonating an individual, there may be scenarios when it is of benefit to others to assume an identity of another service user, think about the field of sport and using someone else's urine samples to pass drug tests. Other examples could be where a person is at risk of cultural or domestic abuse and the abuser prevents a service user from speaking with anyone that may notify emergency or social services by using another person to act as the service user. There sadly could even be instances where a service user has passed away but the carers have not notified the relevant services and are continuing to claim benefits in the deceased person's name and drafted in a willing 'body' to pose as the service user. It sounds extreme and more akin to an article on your local news or chapter from a detective saga (not to mention a lot of effort for the person undertaking the cover up), but if you can imagine it as a scenario there is a possibility it could be reality.

Ultimately, if you are ever in doubt that someone is not who they say they are and you have done all reasonable checks and still feel that there is something not quite right, it is your duty to report your concerns. To the service user, you can politely state that you are unable to access the relevant information and you will contact them to rearrange giving you an opportunity to discuss and share your concerns.

If you have concerns that any abuse is taking place and fear that a service user is in imminent danger, follow your local safeguarding protocols that you would follow. Your organisation may have defined a specific operating procedure for virtual working so please adhere to this wherever relevant. If not, for all other instances, revert to the face-to-face protocols. There are some specific areas of abuse we know have increased (see resources links for information).

In these instances, it may be harder to get a service user alone to ask if they need help, but our duty of care as clinicians remains the same as in any other setting or circumstance and there are ways we may offer support as well as our duty of care to document any concerns and following safeguarding protocols. For further information, see also Chapter 26 for more information around session safety and security.

Even if your assumptions are later revealed to be incorrect and nothing untoward has in fact occurred, you are reassured that you have acted in best interest based on evidence at the time, with the knowledge that, had the concern been valid, you could potentially have prevented or stopped harm occurring or identity fraud.

I SPY WITH MY LITTLE EYE: ESTABLISHING AND MANAGING PARTICIPANTS

How many times have you asked, 'who have you got with you today?' and even when you can hear others or catch a glimpse of someone in the rear of a screen there is sometimes the decline to respond or make fully transparent those who are with them. Although it may seem like a polite and innocent conversation starter, it actually serves a much more onerous and significant purpose in that it forms one of the mechanisms we have for safeguarding our service users. It has been discussed numerous times in terms of,

- How do we really know who we are engaging with when we are in a virtual consultation?
- Do we need to consent and ID check everyone in the room, or just those over certain ages?

There are also concerns of whether persons or carers are recording sessions without the knowledge of the clinician. As with every line of discussion, there are also arguments that, for 'quality control' purposes, persons should be encouraged to record the clinician! Whilst this is likely to pose more IG questions and raise further concerns, there is validity in the premise of this reasoning, as quality reassurance of virtual practice is something that has yet to be developed with any robustness and is currently reliant with a second or senior clinician either being present or 'dialling in' to review the clinician's management of the person and session.

DOI: 10.4324/9781003269724-29

There are numerous ways to authenticate participants and will be dependent on 1:1 or group settings, and these suggestions can be adapted to best fit the circumstances; however, the likelihood is that the less likely you are appearing to be conducting an interview worthy of a courtroom, the more likely you will receive full and frank responses. There are a number of methods you can use to elicit information, including friendly and informal and natural flow of conversation, 'what have you been doing this morning, who is with you today?' If they answer, 'no one', meaning no one is in the room with them, it's always best to clarify if there is anyone else in the house with them in case they turn up mid-session! Advise it's always helpful to know of anyone with them and that you will jot it down in their notes as a record.

The other tack is the more formal route, where it's a deliberate highlighting of who is with them in the room and the house and outlining you are making a record of who was present similar to the outset of an in-person appointment where you would clarify from the outset.

The two styles of eliciting the same information may be used interchangeably and for different purposes or person groups. For example, the informal approach may be more readily tolerated by younger persons or those with anxiety who are finding it difficult to engage. More formal approaches can work really well where it's obvious a person has additional people with them and they haven't volunteered the information as well as with virtual group sessions. This is often forgotten as part of the process as it is overtly assumed the person will be alone but could be attending with a whole room of people behind them in earshot or multiple other persons.

- Clarify the person and their own ID using their health record information (DOB, address is usually sufficient, if any additional concerns and you require further reassurance you can ask them something from their record that only they or a close person would know, like confirming their telephone number, any allergies or perhaps next of kin).

- Clarify formally or informally who else is with them today.
- Ask that they do not use a background so you are able to see anyone that enters the room during the session.
- Consider how you might address any safeguarding concerns you might have about any consultations you undertake where a third party could be a risk to the person or acting as a blocker to care in anyway.
- Remember it's equally as important to document anyone that leaves mid-consultation, even if temporarily and they return. For example, if after they have left you have shared a diagnosis, feedback or information around next steps. Documenting this ensures that any clinical information in the person's record is accurate and, should it be queried at a later point why someone who was in the appointment wasn't part of conversations, there is a record why.

GROUP THERAPY OR DIGITAL PARTY? ESTABLISHING GROUP RULES

Like all virtual consultations, many individuals have very positive experiences of group therapy across many services and it is a method being used across both primary and secondary care to support the self-management of a range of healthcare needs remotely. It can be used to reduce the extent to which one-to-one clinical input is required for a number of individuals in particular. This can have a very positive impact on decreasing service waiting lists as multiple persons, where clinically appropriate, can be offered appointments as part of a group, which also means they can be seen much more quickly than waiting for individual therapy. This method of service redesign and delivery is becoming much more widely used across the NHS with outcomes increasingly reported with positive impact nationally. In speech and language, group therapy isn't uncommon with programmes such as the Lee Silverman Voice Technique (LSVT) offered within a group. However, as an in-person-based intervention, the challenge was how would this translate to online-based therapy, but it did and it does. By keeping groups small, minimising distractions, a therapist and an assistant if possible working in tandem to spot each other can be really helpful for any group setting.

I've had both personal and professional experience of group therapy, which was very different in both instances as I approached them in entirely different ways, although I did find it was difficult to not be 'SLT me', as early on in the use of virtual group clinics and in numerous instances it was evident the parameters for hosting these were undefined. As a result I was drawn to research existing advice for group guidance which was limited in the UK at the time. Instead, I developed my group guidance based on other suggestions I collated and went on to share with a number of colleagues in other organisations regionally and nationally across SLT services and beyond.

These group rules can be downloaded in the resources section as a PDF.

VIDEO GROUP BENEFITS

- As a hugely useful vehicle for mobilising people collectively.
- Sharing a common goal, finding allies in their condition.
- Enable, empower and promote empathy in participants through shared experiences.
- For clinicians it can allow for the same therapy objectives or information to be shared once rather than multiple times.

DRAWBACKS AND CONSIDERATIONS

There are no right or wrong answers to this list! These are considerations collated from discussions and evaluations and are there to prompt your own thoughts and reflections about group therapy.

- Virtual groups may be harder to enforce rules and attendance.
- How will you manage group etiquette?
- Just because an in-person group might be appropriate, does it mean a virtual one is for the same person?
- Can you have the same amount of people in a virtual group as in an in-person group?

Video groups will continue to have valid use in many therapeutic situations, particularly as we align more with the NHS Long Term plans for people to manage their own healthcare more autonomously by engaging with digital tools and remote monitoring means to do this, and group therapy offers a pathway for this. In speech and language it could be effectively used not only as rehab or treatment interventions in adult services, but also as preventative parent or carer skills workshops, and in paediatric and young people's services. Examples of these that are already being offered by NHS and healthcare organisations include autism support (CYGNET and diagnosis Healios), early language skills, makaton, sign and sign or rhythm and rhyme sessions.

It's also an opportunity to collaborate and provide MDT sessions. An MDT doesn't have to be professionals discussing a person, it can be professionals sharing practice and learning, which in turn contributes to CPD but also enables a group of people to receive care collectively across both number and service if these complement each other as a pathway innovation. For example, speech and language therapists and dieticians may collaborate with Macmillan nurses to support head and neck cancer persons. This could reduce the number of appointments both services and citizens need to commit to and provide peer group support networks in one place as an effective means of delivering care in combination.

WHEN SECURITY GETS PERSONAL

The past few chapters have highlighted that digital security and safety are an integral process to providing virtual care to people, and under the umbrella of security there is an abundance of terms and acronyms, from information governance and DPIAs to clinical risk management and CSOs, as well as the plethora of considerations when using digital tools to engage we must be aware of and manage on top of 'the day job'! So let's keep security simple.

DO (TICK)

- Use a blurred background or alternative background where possible.
- If not, remove any family photographs or identifying images, such as new home or our home images that might detail family names.
- Be observant and responsive in your engagement, supporting you building a rapport and safeguarding.

DON'T

- Reveal the location of your home or an organisation or school a member of your family attends (photos might also be indicative of this).
- Allow yourself to feel intimidated in your own home. If ever this is the case, shut down the conversation, ensuring all windows and browsers are closed.

Everyone deserves to feel that they and their identity and information are safe and protected, and we as clinicians are no different. We may be working from our homes in offices,

DOI: 10.4324/9781003269724-31

living rooms, kitchens or bedrooms, but these are our personal spaces and taking a few simple steps to keep them private can really make a difference to the tone of the call, laying boundaries of what is acceptable to share and not, as well as keeping you and your family's information safe. If in doubt, check with a senior clinician, your information governance lead or data protection officer for more advice about your security during consultations.

REMOTE RAPPORT: FOREVER MORE OR NEVERMORE?

ESTABLISHING A RAPPORT

The assumption when remote consultations were discussed initially in many clinical circles was a concern around whether it would ever be possible to establish and maintain the same rapport that we might associate with in-person engagement.

Imagine, if you will, for a moment the world of online dating. An increasing amount of individuals find love online, with a recent study from Stanford University (Rosenfiled, Thomas and Hausen, 2019) indicating that over a fifth of heterosexual couples and almost three times that statistic for gay couples have met online. A similar review of Match Group outcomes, a host of multiple dating applications, suggests a significant increase in registrations in recent months. It seems that those who use online methods for dating are not only using them for convenience and flexibility but are testing the waters and using the medium as a virtual safety net prior to an in-person meeting. What then does this have to do with online consultations? It's all about the connection, the spark or rapport built during these online interactions! If and when these individuals meet in person those awkward first introductions are bypassed and the relationship and conversation can continue from where it was left off, uninhibited and unencumbered by the concerns of how to initiate communication when you 'meet' for the first time.

This rationale extends over to the clinical environment. We can actually start to build the rapport pre-actual consultation with other elements of the digital care pathway, seeking to lower barriers and promote confidence in the clinical process.

104

DOI: 10.4324/9781003269724-32

In a review of video consultations during Covid-19 to compare them to telephone consultations, it was highlighted that being able to see a clinician led to rapport-building being easier (Car, Koh, Foong and Wang, 2020). With the foundations of a rapport initiated, the preliminary support can be used to empower an individual (RCSLT, 2020) through enhancing competences as well as to reassure and encourage, which may play an additional but valuable role, particularly anxious or hesitant service users.

Covert empowerment may feel almost Poirot-esque in nature, but it is a way of ensuring a person is prepared and establishing where support may need focussing before, during or after the virtual interaction. Much of our initial assessments in-person harness the inner investigator in us as we unpick the history to join the dots, but it is important to remember that, whilst the delivery medium we use may be different, the clinical method, processes and interventions are fundamentally the same. These scoping exercises to lead a service user into a new way of working offer a dual purpose, such as to undertake relevant pre-checks, from clarifying devices and sharing security advice to reiterating times, dates or necessary equipment.

There are instances when these pre-checks will be with a service user proxy, such as if the service user is a care home resident or requires third party support to engage with specific assessments (see Chapters 10, 14 and 16).

For those of us who began virtual consultations pre-Covid-19 or very early into the pandemic, it may have initially been the other way around, in that we had already met our persons in-person and were transitioning to virtual care. Meaning at the time of the initial virtual appointment many of the clinical checks, validations of identity and even goal-setting exercises had been completed. These initial sessions would have looked and felt different as these clinicians knew what to expect when interacting with a specific service user in terms of physical features, setting boundaries and managing expectations of the session, based on current and previous engagement and emotional behaviours.

AN EXTRA PAIR OF HANDS:
HCPS AS DIGITAL PARTNERS

Utilising healthcare practitioners in community was unheard of in most SLT communities a relatively short time ago, no more so than in the management of swallow. The thought of not directly assessing a person and the almost ceremonial 'laying on of hands' was almost too much to process and led to concern, anxiety about increased risk. The biggest question being: were there more risks assessing remotely or not assessing until an in-person assessment was possible?

Just before the first wave of the pandemic, my awareness of remote working in the adult speech and language community began to increase, having been introduced to leads working in the remote swallowing space in other areas of the UK following presenting at Microsoft's national healthcare conference. To me, the work that was happening which focussed on training care workers in residential settings to support SLTs during dysphagia assessments delivered remotely was innovative, practical and obvious. I saw the risk, but the benefit of what could be achieved outweighed the negatives that had crossed my mind.

It offered a hybrid opportunity, blending remote digital care from a qualified clinician with that of an upskilled carer in the same room as the person immediately increasing benefit, as not only were they there, they were familiar to the resident being assessed. This was in contrast to face-to-face assessment, whereby a therapist someone had never met before suddenly appears to begin what, for the elderly, aphasic and/or dementia-sufferers could be anxiety-inducing interventions that may lead to withdrawal or refusal though fear of the unknown.

DOI: 10.4324/9781003269724-33

However, across the SLT community, understandably, there continued to be significant anxiety and reluctance about how this would be implemented as a safe practice (including documentation), and how the risks of aspiration would be mitigated.

My research highlighted that two NHS time-served SLTs, RCSLT fellow, lecturer and leading dysphagia management expert, Dr Elizabeth Boaden and her colleague, Digital Clinical Lead Veronica Southern, had developed a method of safely and efficiently providing swallow management, reducing admissions, costs and mortality through creating Teleswallowing LTD. Having already developed and trialled their approach over a six-year period to train staff and support people predominantly in residential care, they progressed the training in response to Covid-19 and the pressures that were being seen on SLTs nationwide. Instead of delivering in-person, whole-day training sessions, the packages have been translated to digital formats available through the training portal Myako, and are a great starting point for increasing whole setting awareness of swallow management as well as targeted training for those supporting SLTs during assessments. In April 2022 they had a pilot approved to use the teleswallowing system across social care settings in Blackpool. Funded by Nestle, supported by the local foundation trust and using the the Docabode platform to manage clinician time and patient flow. The outcomes will be shared. Mapped against the Eating, Drinking and Swallowing Competency Framework (EDSCF), the training programme allows healthcare professionals to undertake aggregated levels of training relevant to the roles they are in within care settings. From support workers to home managers to chefs, acknowledging that dysphagia management is everyone's responsibility is at the core of the programmes, alongside how to identify and mitigate problems that may occur. For those identified as being assessment support, they learn the basics of swallow management, the physiology of the swallow and what to look for in signs and symptoms in order that they efficiently and safely support SLTs to safely undertake dysphagia assessments remotely by being the therapist's 'hands'.

Therapists practising remotely supported by a third party has many benefits, including quicker response times to management, as Healthcare Professionals (HCPs) that have increased awareness also can prevent issues escalating as well as responding when they do arise.

Where SLT's are not routinely visiting, have set days to attend or services are just stretched due to illness, leave or funding, increasing awareness of staff to support swallow management can have other benefits. These include admission prevention, which in turn results in cost savings, but this can also improve quality of life as it means people aren't ricocheting in and out of hospital because they coughed on shepherds pie or apple pie and custard.

The RCSLT has supported a clinical decision-making tool for dysphagia management supported by numerous resources that enable the clinician to not only make the appropriate clinical judgements but to make use of the relevant tools and resources available, including maximising the skills and support of healthcare practitioners.

A TANGLED WEB: BROWSERS
AND WINDOWS

The web can be a dark and shady place to be, especially if you have no idea of the difference between browsers and windows, let alone all the other complexities of tabs, bookmarking, links and so on!

The browser you are using will be dependent on the age and upgrade of the machine and system you are using. It is the software that allows you to access the internet.

Some organisations have particular preferences and you may have to use these by default or change your settings if you would like to use an alternative.

Five browsers you may be most familiar with are,

1. Microsoft Edge – highest overall use in general.
2. Google Chrome – particularly suited to Gmail users.
3. Mozilla Firefox – has heightened internet privacy.
4. Vivaldi – a customisable browser, but is a bit like Microsoft Edge or Chrome with lots of extensions!
5. Apple Safari – only available on Apple operating systems, and most NHS organisations don't use Apple devices.

There are others, Internet Explorer for example still exists, but is being phased-out as it has been replaced with Edge. You may find that certain platforms are restricted by the browsers and you need to 'launch' a particular browser to be able to use some software. However, software companies have begun to acknowledge that they may miss out on both customers and revenue by not making their product available, and so wherever possible it's likely a product will be enabled across as many browsers as possible. The main comparison is usually between Google Chrome, which is often a preferred browser to Safari which may deny or limit access.

Unlike selecting if it will be a round, square or any other shaped window like the days of Playschool and its successors, windows are like digital pages on the internet, also known as tabs.

There are two types of window that you will encounter. The internet variety typically appears across the top of the screen and you might have any amount open at any one time, although I've learned that less is definitely more where these are concerned and accidents can and do happen the more you have open.

Applications or files windows are usually those which you see icons for across your task bar along the bottom of the screen. For example, the internet browser, Word and folders or files from your device.

Managing Windows/tabs during a session is relatively straightforward and comes down to the three Rs.

1. Record and Record – make sure you only have the person's record you are seeing at the time or waiting to join a call open, and ensure that you record everything you need to before opening another.
2. Resources – have the windows/tabs open for any online resources or files on your device.
3. Ruthless – don't have things open just because you think you might need them, close them down. This is not about *not* being prepared but about streamlining what you need to do and what you are likely to need during a session.

To close Windows/tabs down, just click the cross in the right-hand corner of the tab on internet or select 'close window' in the dropdown options across the bottom of the screen. You will need your platform open too so you can join the call, I'm sure there will be instances of actually forgetting to open the link and wondering why you are all alone until you realise why!

32

CLOSING CONVERSATIONS

It might sound obvious but ending a conversation is just as important as how we start and manage a conversation. Chapter 31 highlights some general advice for shutting down a conversation, but do we need to use different language in virtual consultations than we would in person?

In short, the answer is no, we don't need to change what we say, but how we say, use and direct language is slightly different as we have to be more overt to ensure that the message has been received as intended and may require a little extra by way of check-in than in an in-person appointment.

We also have to clarify timescales more directly than in-person appointments as it can be much harder to claw back time from back-to-back virtual appointments than delivering them from a clinic room where set sessions map out the day and we don't succumb as easily to skipping breaks to get through the work loads.

Recounting and reviewing the session at junctures (these will feel sensible times to check in, perhaps after a new exercise has been explained or you are reviewing a previous one. Ensure that whilst you are in sync you are actually 'insync'! Using these as the opportunity you need to check that the goals, expectations and boundaries set have been accepted and understood. Again, record in the electronic record any salient points of reference that may later be revisited.

- The most important aspects when closing a session are that you have done it safely.
- Any outstanding discussions, aims and objectives are documented to follow up in the next session.

DOI: 10.4324/9781003269724-35

- The person feels they have received the same quality and level of care they would have had they attended in person.
- If you are able to follow up with an electronic feedback form this is a good way to support internal service evaluations and can also support short- and long-term data collections specific to virtual consultations for regional or national research, too.

33

SHUTDOWN: ENDING A REMOTE CONSULTATION SAFELY

As we draw near to the close of a consultation, just as in everything we do, there will be our own way of approaching. So, when it comes to ending a remote consultation, what is the best way to bring the session to an end?

I have just two words to do this. *Safely* and *efficiently*. My advice is do all things as efficiently as possible, but ensure that, whatever you do, it is above all as safe as possible for both you and the individual or group you are working with. In time, you should be able to do these with minimum effort as they will become part of your,

- Shutdown
- Write up
- Log off
- Sign out

Why? Have you ever had the 'have I left the oven on' feeling? This is a similar feeling to 'have I closed the session down properly', although instead of your jacket potatoes frazzling to a lump of charcoal, not closing a session properly can lead to security breaches. Being certain about whether you have safely closed a platform window, i.e. the one that is hosting a consultation, is important. Checking everything is metaphorically wiped down and sterilised before resetting for the next session is a useful analogy to have, so think of closing windows as this sort of refresh process between consultations.

An extreme example, and I'm only aware of it happening once where this process wasn't done effectively, resulted in two individuals having their virtual consult windows open in tandem. On this occasion, instead of closing the window the clinician only minimised it, meaning that the other person, while couldn't see or be seen, could hear what was happening in the other person's consultation! They reported this very quickly and allowed the situation to be dealt with and investigated, but it does really validate why the closing down process is such a vital one.

So, to avoid any security slip ups as you near the finishing line, there are a number of things it's really useful to remember, just as you do when you finish a session in person.

- Summarise the goals set in the session: clarify where these have been recorded and, if a copy of these will be shared with the person, check you have their email address or mobile number to send an attachment.
- Agree your next appointment: if possible, book it, if not, highlight the process and set expectations, such as when they will receive their appointment time and date and via what means.
- Recap what you will do between sessions: referrals, resources, etc.
- Recap how you can be contacted and set expectations for responses: outline that electronic response times (email, SMS, portal, if relevant) are the same as your standard service response times.
- Before you open up another person's record, finish the notes you are writing to avoid writing Mr Smith's session up in Miss Smyth's record!

TOP TIP: It is worth checking if they are happy to have appointment sent in the same way, e.g. if it was email previously, is that still OK, or has something changed so you can avoid the 'I didn't get my appointment' chat?

- End on time: it's easy for time to run away. A useful strategy is to set a timer on your phone for ten minutes before the end of the session. Make a point of saying, 'we only have ten minutes left, before we end I need to let you know X, Y, Z and then we will have a few minutes if you have any questions'.

- If the session doesn't come to a natural end, unless it warrants a clinical or safeguarding response immediately, advise that you have made a note to pick it up at the next session but you are really sorry your next appointment is in the waiting room … even if the platform you are using doesn't have one!

- Finally: close everything down so you start your next session with the right record and relevant tabs open.

THE REMOTE TOOLS: CREATING A DIGITAL TOOLKIT

ACCESSIBILITY: WINDOWS AND YOU!

I have been hugely fortunate to have worked with some of the most passionate leads in the technology sector full stop. It is has been even more exciting to see how industry giants have used their insight and innovation to support not just health-care and digital transformation on a grand scale but focussed their attention on digital accessibility and inclusion across this sector. As a clinician positioned within the NHS I have been enormously privileged to harness and absorb the brilliance, passion, dedication and determination of these individuals who are supporting developments and innovations that not only benefit everyday life but, can positively impact in healthcare delivery too. As a parent and advocate of individuals with dis-abilities and as a neurodiverse individual, this is something which has become increasingly important in the work I do, and understanding how I can support others has been a journey of discovery, not least because I found that there is so much at our fingertips … literally!

Did you know that the keys underneath your fingers that you type on every single day on your phone, your tablet, laptop or desktop don't just type letters and numbers, but many also function as part of a series of increasingly sophisticated inbuilt accessibility features created to enhance everyday activities and make daily tasks easier. Many were developed in response to meeting a specific accessibility need and have been found to have wider-reaching benefits for others. It could be the smallest or the simplest of changes that have the most impact.

There are some we take for granted and don't even recog-nise as accessibility tools, they are just features of our ever-advancing and technologically enabled devices. Features such

DOI: 10.4324/9781003269724-38

as changing and enlarging the font, we might do it because we like a particular style, but have never thought about it being more accessible, it's just easier to read; but do you know the ones that can make reading easier for individuals with visual impairment or dyslexia? The OpenDyslexic font was created by American Abelardo Gonzalez and released as a free and open source font in 2011.

San Serif fonts such as Arial and the ever-popular Comic Sans, are less visually crowded and so can make it slightly easier to read despite having heard by colleagues in education, 'if I ever see Comic Sans again …' Although it's typically teachers, so SLTs may not have such intensity of feeling. Other fonts which may be dyslexia-friendly alternatives include,

- Verdana
- Century Gothic
- Trebuchet
- Calibri
- Open Sans

Font size is recommended to be 12–14 point, although if you are working in an alternate provision or education setting, staff may require this to be larger depending on the individual. For visually impaired individuals, this is determined by the severity of their sight but, as a rule, the darker and larger the font, the easier it makes the visibility and clarity, so it can make a big difference to some.

Where do you find these magical buttons of accessibility joy? Right in front of you! While this chapter is largely relevant to those who will access a Windows device at some point during their working day, there are lots of accessibility tools and add-ons that can be found on most devices now by searching the accessibility settings on the device.

Alternatively, there are lots of specific pieces of software for almost every challenge with many programmes focussed around translating speech to text as well as app versions of familiar programmes with accessibility solutions built-in, such as Microsoft Word.

As many clinicians will use a laptop or desktop with keyboard, the following tips are focussed on the accessibility functions that are accessed by making physical changes with keys or in the accessibility menu.

The Windows key – it looks like a four-square window and can sometimes be found between Ctrl and Alt, or in a similar position to the left of the space bar (Figure 34.1).

This button of four-square plus U, as in Windows + U (you), allegedly because it comes from the personalisation element of functions, opens the world to a whole host of features and functions that can tailor your experience, but you can also maximise their value for those you work with synchronously (live) or asynchronously (outside of the session).

The alternative way to find your way to access these features is simply to search 'Accessibility' in the search bar (Windows 11). This has recently been updated from other versions, having previously been referred to as Ease of Access. The operating system you are accessing may affect the features and experiences you are able to interact and engage with. The update is a result of disability community co-designing the new iteration and having highlighted that simply referring to accessibility was much clearer. It's also much easier to actually access with a clearer icon that the developers have identified simply as 'human', representing individual personalisation.

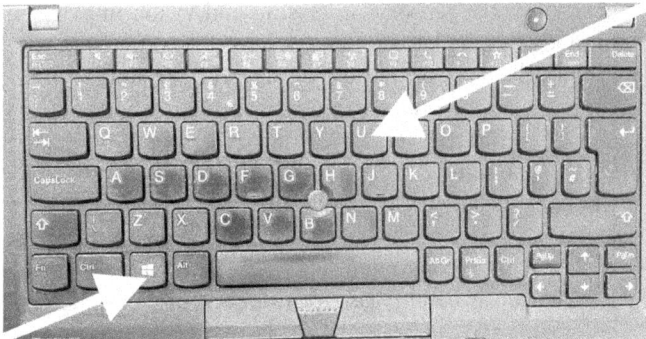

Figure 34.1 Keyboard

To make it even easier to select features and personalise a device, the option is also within both log in and off screens.

There are new and updated features in the most recent version utilising the most cutting-edge technology to minimise exclusion of access and maximise success and engagement. One significant update is 'Windows Voice Typing', a highly sensitive and powerful speech-to-text tool that is designed for people who have a vast number of reasons to 'write with their voice' (Microsoft Blog, October 2021 – see resources for full article and further information).

Not all features are relevant to everyone, but accessibility tools can not only improve your professional experience, making tasks easier and quicker to complete, but may benefit your personal experience, visual and auditory comfort, physical experience where injury or disability or difference may impact the length of time, pace of work and comfort of using a device. Finally, it can offer you a method to support individuals you work with in therapy to maximise their own engagement by suggesting small changes that may make a big difference to their communicative interactions and experiences.

So, let's start at the beginning and get personal.

Once you are in the Accessibility/Ease of Access menu, you can start to make changes and amendments to your user experience (UX) such as,

- Change polarity/contrast – individuals with colour blindness, dyslexia, sensory processing and vision impairment individuals may benefit from this feature.
- Nightlight – I have this set to daylight hours so the contrast auto changes to a warmer light as the daylight changes and reduces glare and over stimulation from white/blue light.
- Changes include background colour, like overlays for dyslexia; the colour of the background can make a difference.
- Mouse pointer colour and size.
- Keyboard can be changed to include symbols – these are emoticons and can be used to replace words in text in applications such as Word and PowerPoint.

Clinicians quite literally in their hundreds and thousands have accessed Microsoft Teams now, which seems so strange as we almost take for granted this powerful therapy tool, and yet when I started my Teams journey in 2017, this was most definitely not the case. Organisations were becoming familiar with it for corporate and administrative use, but it was an underused method of clinical engagement in the UK until the immersion into a global pandemic.

Microsoft Teams as a platform, like many of the other suites of tools within Office 365, has numerous features that really support great clinical engagement. There are literally 100s if not 1000s of applications (apps) available directly through Teams. It's worth noting that you may have limited access or not be able to download these depending on your organisation's IG policies and your Microsoft Licence, which may be different depending on your role within an organisation and related to cost. The apps cover everything from online whiteboards and collaborative document writing to supporting interaction and accessibility of speech, be it blurring the background, a tool originally designed to minimise visual disturbance and make it easier to lip read, through to closed caption and transcription or translation of whole conversations.

One question that has been raised through SLT forums and several national workshops is the challenge raised by engaging a translator. With the dynamic reported consistently as being changed and the practicalities of the link being shared with someone who is neither patient, carer or clinician, it's been an area of much discussion and, at times, frustration. Using digital tools to support this can really maximise the session and reduce the stress on patients and clinicians as the process is automatic and is generated from speech dictation – speech-to-text.

TRANSLATOR

CONVERSATIONS – MICROSOFT TRANSLATOR

Using Microsoft Teams and Microsoft Translator to host a multilingual meeting can be a useful tool to draw on e.g. between home, school and clinician so parent/carer is able to speak in first language which is translated synchronously for other participants.

Several options are available and links to find out more, including how to download and use Microsoft Translator, can be found in the online resources section.

Translation tools as a method of supporting engagement in therapy or meetings, at face value allows multiple people to participate in a Teams call in their preferred language, but this also provides accessibility, reduces additional barriers and supports empowerment and equality for individuals, so the interaction and content of information gathered is the focus, rather than the logistical challenge of conversing with an individual in a different language may pose. This can also support reducing misinterpretation of information that may be clinically relevant and provide autonomy and confidence for those you are working with.

Additionally, the transcription feature can be used to capture the typed or spoken word and is recorded and has the potential to be shared after the meeting ends.

As with Microsoft Translator, TranslateIt and Realtime Translator are just two apps available in Teams to support those where languages spoken may be different to those in meeting/appointment. These will be added to as more partners onboard their tools. Translation apps and more can be searched for within Teams under apps.

TRANSCRIPTION – AVAILABLE IN TEAMS

The transcription will be made available within the chat and a copy will be recorded and stored. Please make sure that anyone that is participating is aware that this feature has been instigated in the same way you would if recording.

To translate in a document, right click and select the Translate option that will appear on the list and a box will appear in the right-hand side of the screen. Highlight the text and change the language you would like this to be in!

LIVE CAPTIONS

To utilise this feature during a Teams meeting, once in a call, select the three dots from the tool bar.

READING PREFERENCES

We briefly visited tools to support individuals where reading text may be a barrier so the reading preferences tool kit, which can be found in several of the Microsoft applications, including Word, PowerPoint and OneNote, can make a huge difference.

Creating accessible documents is a skill that is invaluable not just for speech and language therapists but one all clinicians and individuals working in healthcare support roles would benefit from an awareness of. There are some great 'how-to' online resources from various organisations, including Microsoft, which can easily be found online. Some of these have been included in the resources section.

This tool is not only great for clinicians that want to make use of speech-to-text features, but it can be a really useful set of tools to signpost different patient groups to for different reasons.

The Immersive Reader tool is accessed from the tool bar across the top of the page within an open document. Open 'View' and the select 'Immersive Reader'. Select Immersive Reader and from here you can choose,

- Background colour.
- Break text down into syllables.
- Increase spacing between words and columns (tracking).
- Highlight a specific line to focus the reader. This is particularly useful for individuals with dyslexia, for example.
- You can also select 'Read Aloud' for the whole document or highlighted selection in the same tool bar.

Remember, the Immersive Reader function needs to be closed using the red cross to return to standard functions or you won't be able to return to other standard features or navigate the document.

The Immersive Reader function is available in most of the Office 365 products and is a feature of certain websites. The BBC News website is a good example of this and can be found wherever the Immersive Reader icon is .

You can select from three voices to be read to by, one male and two females, George, Susan and Hazel. These can be selected from the main sounds function page (search sounds in the search bar to change).

DICTATE

The opposite function to Immersive Reader and Read Aloud functions, where the feature relies on what is already documented, instead Dictate will allow for individuals to do just that: they will be able to speak what they want to say instead of type. This is particularly useful for individuals that have mobility or dexterity problems, such as those who need an alternative to typing. It allows for an individual to remain autonomous and independent. You do have to be very prescriptive and ensure that capital letters and full stops (a little like a consultant dictating a letter) are in the right place, but in general it's a very accurate method of dictating and transcribing perhaps letters, documents, medical reports, etc., as this exercise shows because I dictated it!

You can also dictate in multiple languages.

If, for example, I was a Spanish speaker, I could change the language to reflect this by selecting Spanish as my spoken language, enabling me to speak in my preferred language. It will then dictate and represent in this language within the document, e.g. 'How are you', '*Cómo está*'.

'*Dushenka*' (soul) in Russian is represented by Russian graphemes Доченька.

Or '*Sayonara*' (goodbye) in Japanese is represented by the symbolsヽ さよなら.

There are some limitations to the languages available, such as dialects within a language, as it tends to generalise, so it may be that using an alternative translation method such as a subsequent web tool or app that you can copy and paste from is more efficient and accurate depending on purpose and need. However, it is worth considering for quick translations to support sessions. For example, pre-prepared session guidance to support therapy exercises so a parent can help their child.

CHROME/EDGE – IMMERSIVE READER

Many websites, particularly high-profile and corporate web-sites such as BBC News utilise the accessibility features of Immersive Reader. Here you can have the document read aloud to you, break it up in a similar way to make it easier to read and can also make use of the Boardmaker picture dictionary. This is a picture/symbol system well known in the communication world and often associated with those who have receptive and/or expressive language challenges. It can also be useful to highlight abstract concepts utilising a visual image to support written or spoken word. Typically the Boardmaker images available in Office 365 products are common nouns or verbs, so don't expect there is a picture representation for every word, it doesn't quite work like that!

If you imagine the rhebus stories you may have encountered at school where every so often a word is missing and you fill it in by selecting the right picture to make the story or passage make sense, that is the principle the picture dictionary utilises.

Advanced uses of this can be cutting and pasting the images seen to create documents, stories or resources so images are consistent. This is useful if you are working with individuals that respond well to familiarity.

POWERPOINT

There are some great features hiding in PowerPoint that enable you to create resources dynamically using the AI capabilities within the software. This may include using the design generator to create simple visual resources!

By typing or using the 'Dictate' function for the target word into a slide, and using the design generator to represent simple concepts such as animals, you can quickly and easily create meaningful documents and resources to share with individuals that can be tailored to them personally for a variety of reasons. There are increased accessibility functions specifically in PowerPoint with the Accessibility Ribbon. It uses inbuilt AI to check your presentation slides to ensure they are maximally accessible. For example, are they easy to read, could images have been included, could headings have been included? (as well as the function to now include subtitles or live captions as you present).

Another function that is underused and could be really utilised for so many purposes in both adult and paediatric therapy, is embedding a thumbnail video for sign language (BSL or Makaton) and lip reading feature. This has recently been updated and received a name in its own right, 'Cameo', within PowerPoint and other Office 365 tools. It allows for the video to be positioned wherever the user wants as well as offering slide design/layout suggestions for optimal viewing.

ONLINE TRAINING

There is an abundance of online training and resourcing available around making electronic documents more accessible, and of course Microsoft have produced their own open access training which is free and offers a host of tips, tricks and suggestions for getting the most out of what you already have to work with.

For many employers this will be a bonus, as training and CPD packages can be costly and expensive as well as rapidly going out of date.

Microsoft are one of many companies that have developed accessibility resources but, having engaged with the team on a number of projects, they are really passionate about making change and the team behind the tools are people with life experiences that really 'get' the challenges that can occur. From both a professional and a personal perspective, the support that is available is extensive and the one thing I found frustrating above everything else was no one knew that this existed.

Technical support for customers with accessibility needs are a focus and there is dedicated help via the Microsoft Disability Answer Desk. The team are trained in multiple assistive technologies, speak English, French and Spanish and Sign Language. This is a really useful tool for signposting people you are supporting to personalise their user experiences, enhance resources and therapy interventions and increase confidence in digital skills.

For professionals, commercial or enterprise users there is an alternative option via the enterprise Disability help desk.

This areas is VAST and in one chapter alone I can barely scratch the surface or do it the justice it rightly deserves. These features are updated regularly with more accessibility features being added than ever. With each new update and version new features will be developed and more will become possible!

For even more information, including the links to the Microsoft Accessibility website, training modules, information targeted to creating accessible documents for a range of individuals and the links for the help desk offer, the online resources have a list of relevant links.

35

THE BARE ACCESSIBLES

Apps and wearable devices are becoming more embedded in our health and care pathways and the expectation is that individuals will be more autonomous in managing their own healthcare. Wearables range from simple pedometers and mainstream smartwatches that track general fitness levels to pulse oximetry, apps and websites that manage therapy goals. There are more than 80,000 apps available in the digital healthcare space!

Not all of these are assured, in fact a very small percentage of these are clinically assured as tools that are safe and secure to prescribe to patients as part of their care and even fewer of them are classed as accessible. This is a regulatory requirement of all apps and websites as of June 2021. You can find much more information at Orchahealth.com and for updated current statistics.

GUIDANCE FOR ACCESSIBILITY OF APPS AND WEBSITES

WCAG – WEBSITE CONTENT ACCESSIBILITY GUIDELINES

These are specific guidelines (known as WCAG 2.1) and are an internationally recognised set of recommendations for improving web accessibility. They are a legal requirement of websites and similar guidelines will also impact the development of apps.

They explain how to make digital services, websites and apps accessible to everyone, including users with impairments to their,

- Vision – like severely sight impaired (blind), sight impaired (partially sighted) or colour blind people.

DOI: 10.4324/9781003269724-39

- Hearing - like people who are deaf or hard of hearing.
- Mobility – like those who find it difficult to use a mouse or keyboard.
- Thinking and understanding – like people with dyslexia, autism or learning difficulties.

TESTING FOR ACCESSIBILITY

UNDERSTANDING WCAG 2.1 – SERVICE MANUAL – GOV.UK (WWW.GOV.UK)

If you are using a website or web-hosted application, you can use the link below to test the accessibility of the site. It might seem a strange thing to do, but would you use an assessment that hadn't been checked out for ease of use? A similar function is available within Office 365 documents to enable you to check how accessible a document or resource that you create is and how you can improve it, which is a really easy way of checking that documents and resources that you produce for individuals or groups are as accessible as possible.

www.gov.uk/service-manual/technology/testing-for-accessibility

Accessibility regulations mean public sector organisations have a legal duty to make sure their websites and mobile applications meet accessibility requirements.

Public sector websites must now be accessible and publish an accessibility statement.

Mobile apps have been required to meet the WCAG accessibility regulations since 23 June 2021. The links to these can be found in the resources or below at the following web addresses:

https://accessibility.campaign.gov.uk/
https://accessibilityinsights.io/en/downloads/

Accessibility and inclusion of digital pathways should be 'built in not bolted on', a phrase I often use to highlight that this should not be done retrospectively as an afterthought, or perhaps where the solution is 'an accessible version'. If individuals have access to a product or service then this same product or service should be accessible to everyone. This should be regardless of the impacting factors. We all have a right and deserve to be able to access healthcare in a way that is relevant and meaningful to us.

The tools in this section can go some small way to supporting and recognising what is needed to achieve digital accessibility through design but it is one small part of a very large engine that needs to work collaboratively across many areas to ensure this continues to progress.

WCAG does not assure an app for clinical use, it only supports and reviews the accessibility of the content. For clinical assurance of apps, see Chapter 37.

YOU, ME AND ASD

36

It might sound like the title of a documentary, but there is a real purpose to this section and, as the header suggests, it's not a one-way street. It's no secret that I love virtual consultations for many reasons but, as a patient, they have been enormously beneficial for me, and I'm aware of other neurodiverse individuals who report the same. As yet, NICE (2021) suggests there is limited evidence about the impact of the pandemic on autism services and virtual care, but there are numerous studies including research undertaken by Swansea University Medical School around the positive impact telehealth can have on waiting times for diagnosis. The study was focussed on the adult population and Alfuraydan et al. (2020) suggest that, whilst this is still a limited field, 'there is potential for telehealth methods to improve access to assessment and diagnosis of ASD used in conjunction with existing methods, especially for those with clear autism traits and adults with ASD'. Similar outcomes have been seen in the paediatric field, with several organisations now specialising in remote multidisciplinary diagnosis of autism for children. These pathways have successfully been used in conjunction with existing traditional methods to reduce the time between referrals and diagnosis. More information regarding remote autism diagnosis can be found in the resources section.

Informal reports and blogs indicate the benefits of utilising virtual care including flexibility, not having to attend in-person and sit in unfamiliar surroundings, increased involvement from parents or family and better access to services including speech and language.

Multiple perspectives and experiences are brought to every video consultation but, when neurodiversity is part of that experience, there are a few additional considerations that may make the scenario a little less stressful for those who are engaged in the consultation. As a neurodiverse clinician, patient and parent I have assumed a number of roles during consultations and have developed a series of strategies for managing different circumstances to make the consultation as least stressful as possible as well as remaining professional and calm.

The question is how can we make video consultations more accessible and comfortable for neurodiverse individuals? There are a few really simple suggestions and some of them cross over with the basic advice around setting up your virtual consult scenario outlined in Section 2, but I'll highlight the rationale why these can make a bigger difference to those that function neuro-uniquely.

1. Introduce yourself – we do this almost automatically, but with those with a neurodiversity, this initial introduction can really make or break an encounter. Particularly if any changes in the appointment have occurred (see 4 and 5 of these suggestions)

2. Minimal backgrounds – limiting the visual noise on screen in terms of what is behind you can make a huge difference. In previous chapters this has been discussed in relation to safety and not identifying yourself or your family, but actually a 'quiet' or minimalist background can be much less distracting and in turn reduce anxiety. For example, if you are based in an office or clinic that has shelves full of books and assessments, these can be really off-putting for someone who has difficulty attending and may become fixed instead on the title of a book, counting how many texts there are, focus on a Post-It note sticking out or wondering why the texts aren't alphabetical and size-ordered. Just by blurring the background or having a very plain organisational-branded one (white or black plus the organisation logo are often the least distracting) can make the experience easier from the outset.

3. Annoying or unseen sounds – like having visual distractors, audible ones can be just as challenging for someone. They could even impact assessments of auditory skills if they are loud enough to interfere. The tick of a clock, for example, if it's a particularly loud mechanism, dripping tap, keyboard being hit or chair squeaking. Some of these may be unavoidable, but wherever possible limit noises that are not part of the session, and if you can't, try and limit attention on them by muting yourself when they are talking so they aren't working over the top of the noise.

4. Remove unknown factors where possible – prior to the session it's likely you or if you are really lucky a team admin will have sent out the appointment time, date and who the appointment is with, but that's all they have. This can be really daunting for someone with a neurodiversity, who has increased anxiety because they have limited control over a number of factors, including that it may be the first time they are seeing a clinician and don't know what to expect about the person they will see when they log onto the session. If possible, include a headshot of yourself in the information you send out.

    This may be,

    a. Included within the PDF of the appointment letter attached to SMS or email.

    b. A photo of yourself attached to your work email account that the individual has been able to look at when receiving their appointment information.

    c. Your image on the services web page and include a link to this within the appointment letter so the individual can choose to look up your photo ahead of the appointment.

5. If there is a change, let people know – knowing who you are seeing can be a big part of the increased anxiety for many individuals with a neurodiversity and I have lived experience of changes to clinician without prior knowledge preventing an appointment going ahead due to the individual withdrawing as a result of extreme anxiety.

Not because the clinician was awful, not able to do exactly the same interventions and support a particular individual as the one they were originally seeing, but simply because they weren't expecting to see that person and they had not been updated. With the right communication, everyone will understand that circumstances change, but it can be really hard to adjust to what is already an atypical scenario.

6. Try to limit small talk – we often use general chat to informally cue ourselves into a session, find out about someone's week, morning, etc. We may ask indirect questions that appear to be informal but are for security purposes, e.g. to find out about the people in the house. For someone with a neurodiversity, these may seem inconsequential and unnecessary questions and cause more anxiety as they try and work out why these are being asked. It may be less stressful for them to ask directly and give a reason for the question to be clear and transparent as reducing the element of the unknown, even in our conversations, can have a huge impact. It means they won't spend the rest of the session thinking, 'why did they want to know if I had any pets/been out today/if anyone is due to visit me, etc.'

These suggestions are by no means exhaustive and are strategies that might not work for everyone, if you have met one autistic person, you have met one autistic person, so the anecdote goes. The use of them, however, may work for the individuals you are working with and you should include the individual in any adjustments you make by asking them what works for them. Many people with a neurodiversity will be able to express what makes things harder in unfamiliar contexts such as video appointments, even if they can't express what might make it easier. It's the clinician's ability to take these factors onboard and tailor to the needs of the individual that will make the difference.

You may have ways of making your virtual sessions more autism-friendly. Just because they may sound obvious or simple doesn't necessarily mean someone else will think about it, especially if they haven't had an experience that has called for them to reflect and adapt their usual session management. We often assume that we aren't the expert and everyone will know what we know, but don't be afraid to share your ideas, I guarantee there will be someone that appreciates your insight.

SEEKING APP-ROVAL

There are numerous applications, or what we most commonly refer to as apps, that can provide us with what are termed 'immersive experiences'. Technology that puts us in the picture and provides those who interact with it a mixed-reality platform to engage with.

Developments are happening throughout healthcare, from large-scale virtual reality (VR) innovations with examples that are changing the landscape of healthcare, including remote surgery interventions allowing specialists from across the globe to collaborate, to GPs using VR goggles to remotely assess patients in care homes and advise nursing professionals (yes really!). There are also technologies to support and enhance our everyday experiences and enable improved healthcare outcomes, designed as accessibility tools but with the ability to apply to anyone.

Apps are one element of providing immersive experiences at an easily accessible level. Using just smart phones or tablets, they are readily downloadable and available to cover 100s of areas. Musculoskeletal therapies (MSK), for example, have seen significant growth in this area to support individuals post-operatively for common procedures such as hip and knee replacements, using both synchronous and asynchronous methods to support and manage recovery.

There are apps specific to our own discipline that support all areas, from managing dysphagia to voice and everything in between.

These change all the time and it can be hard to know if they are safe, secure or regulated. Just because something looks nice in the app stores and has five stars doesn't mean it has been approved or is supported by any regulatory body.

We wouldn't use an assessment that we knew nothing about or had not been approved for use, so the same caution should

138   DOI: 10.4324/9781003269724-41

be displayed when considering using digital tools to support therapy.

There are vast libraries of apps that can be prescribed to patients in addition to or as alternatives to medications or other medical or therapeutic interventions. The NHS app library has been a repository over the past few years but this is relatively limited. There is a disclaimer around the use of the apps on the NHS Apps libraries web page to highlight that, whilst listed as assured and approved, they are not managed, owned or updated by anyone within NHS organisations, they are solely the supplier's responsibility. The disclaimer can be found in the resources section.

ORCHA is a widely recognised and growing agency that supports the NHS in assessing and assuring apps for use in healthcare that can be used to enhance therapy and interventions between clinical appointments, as well as to support autonomous management and allow the individual to be their own agent of change.

There are alternatives to this via individual organisations or healthcare systems working with ORCHA to produce specific libraries of apps for specific pathways. This ensures that every app held within ORCHA's library is assured and enables safe and scalable adoption of digital health solutions. ORCHA also supports suppliers to become compliant with the NHS national standards of the Digital Technology Assessment Criteria (DTAC), enabling clinicians and individuals using these tools to be reassured that they have been rigorously reviewed and approved.

REMEMBER – CRCR – CAUTION, RESEARCH, CHECK AND REVIEW!

Do have Caution – don't take an app at face value. Just because it says it is a complete dysphagia therapy tool or a safe and secure method of tracking phonology goals doesn't mean it is! You or the individuals you are working with could be providing all sorts of information to all sorts of people under the guise of swallow management when really it's sucking your data!

Do Research – search the name of the app on the internet, is it recognised, recommended and reliable?

Do Check – discuss with colleagues, it may be that someone else has already trialled an app for the same purpose and can share their insight.

Do Review – don't launch an app on your caseload before you are sure it is safe, secure and fits the purpose you intended. In many trusts, the process of undertaking a Clinical Safety Report is necessary for large-scale implementations or if a new product is at a cost but the smaller interventions and the 'it's just an app' methodology can mean that the same scrutiny isn't applied to the use of the tool. It may sound extreme, but this process of reviewing and checking is really important for assurance and governance. For example, if an app that requires personal information to be added, and it's been managed by the department with individuals accessing their own profile and a data breach occurred because the app's security hadn't been assessed and approved by the information governance and clinical safety teams are not aware of the existence of the tool, there may be no process in place to protect or mitigate, this could have negative implications on several levels. It is always safer to do the due diligence first. It might take longer, but it means there is assurance of safety and security.

WHAT IF WE DON'T HAVE TIME TO DO THIS?

This is where the app libraries and ORCHA might be better placed to be of support. They can help and advise you, not only on speciality-specific apps, and amongst their services they can provide guidance to aid in reducing the unknowns around using and prescribing digital tools, signposting to clinically safe, secure and assured apps and allowing for quicker adoption and implementation, especially where you may be considering multiple apps or larger-scale use of these tools. See the resources section for relevant links to the NHS Library and ORCHA for further information on their web pages.

Ultimately, whatever method you use for selecting and app-roving,

Check It, Don't Chance It!

EMOTIONALLY SPEAKING: USING EMOTICONS TO ENHANCE THERAPY AND OTHER DIGITAL ENGAGEMENT TOOLS IN THERAPY

Open up your messages and look at your most used emoticons, mine are currently a screaming face, a koala and a rainbow! Make of that what you will, but despite us being more familiar with emoticons for sending a cheeky wink or a thumbs up, we can actually use them in therapy because we are already using them in subjective assessments and scales on paper-based assessments, so it takes very little to transfer them to an online version and make use of these visual and globally recognised symbols for therapy purposes.

One really easy example is using a Likert scale to cue an individual in at the start of the session.

By popping up a simple scale of five faces, screen sharing and then giving presenter rights, you can see the other person's cursor and see where they are pointing.

It's great for non-verbal interaction or gently building up to verbal exchanges if you have a slightly reluctant or shy individual that needs a little longer to engage verbally. I have used a similar scale to revert back to and check in for feedback at various points through the session to check that someone is feeling happy with how the session is, that they have understood the activity and then feedback at end of the session (Figure 38.1).

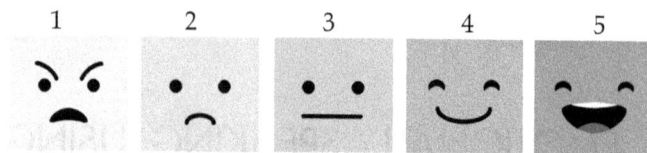

Figure 38.1 Likert scale

If I'm recording in the notes I'll record as numbers rather than describe the face, so I can ask the same questions during subsequent sessions and gauge progression of different parameters using subjective questioning, either as ice breakers or as part of informal assessment and feedback.

It's also useful to be consistent with the style, so if you choose a particular set of faces, try and stick with those as it can be distracting for some if you change even small details such as this and it might be this that becomes the focus of the task rather than the line of questioning you intend!

There are loads of other digital tools that you can use to complement your online sessions that you can bring into your virtual sessions, everything from timers to online quizzes and bubble popping, there's an activity for most eventualities now!

TIMERS

These can be particularly useful for a whole set of reasons. As a voice therapist, one of the main uses I have for timers are to manage breath control and compare this to previous sessions. Yes, you can absolutely use phones with ease, but having it on-screen gives the individual you are working with a visual prompt and incentive, just like they would get if they were with you in the room with a stop watch, and can be a powerful tool for eking out an extra second or two for them to achieve their own personal bests.

They can also be useful for regulating breathing in exercises, such as Lax Vox, for example.

WHITEBOARDS

A fantastic collaboration tool and one which can have multiple uses. They can be used with a varying range of individuals, from paediatrics through to geriatrics depending on the need, objective and information being shared or received. It may be a way of the individual sharing information visually with you as much as you with them.

A practical example of where I have used digital whiteboards has been to pinpoint where an individual's specific difficulty is from a physiological perspective by drawing or annotating images of the larynx. In a clinic, 'Fred The Head' might have been my go-to, but there are a number of reasons this doesn't translate to virtual.

He's clinic-based and I don't have my own personal Fred at home.

It might not translate quite so well to be dissecting a plastic head on-screen as the parts are not easy to see and Fred, despite being only a head, is heavy! He's not easy to hold up and show the camera various body parts whilst tipping to the right angle.

So, having the whiteboard set up with some images you can refer to and highlight as well as also allow for the individual to add any of their own annotations to, point out where they are experiencing pain, discomfort or other symptoms, using the option by way of the cursor to give control to them can be a really useful tool. It allows the individual to feel engaged, heard and in control. Depending on the context, two digital tools could be used in tandem with whiteboards, used in conjunction with emoticons. For example, if working with an aphasic patient that has reduced expressive capacity, these two strategies together could support an individual to independently express some of the more complex ideas without feeling overtly frustrated and unable to communicate or rely on someone else.

ONLINE GAMES

There are multiples sites for online games that have everything from minimal pairs through to prepositions and, just as we would in-person, these activities can be weaved into virtual sessions depending on the individual and therapy objective. Some activities will be more appropriate for younger audiences where some could be adapted for wider groups across more varied age groups and cognitive abilities. My intention is not to promote any one site over another, but there are some links in the resources you may find useful as a starting point if you are looking for ideas to begin with.

ONLINE FLASH CARDS

A tool that is really useful for very structured sessions and keeping things on task. They may be particularly useful if coordinating a group session where you have group objectives, have broken off into breakouts and had smaller discussions happening and then come back together, or to act as prompt cards to encourage group members to contribute.

They are great for language-based activities for instruction-based games or directions. I trained for Lego Therapy several years ago, and although the premise is collaborative and fosters social communication, the format could be done remotely using some clear instructions and a set of flash cards to define the roles of the participants and their tasks to build.

There are sets of templates that can be used so a session can be built quickly and easily as well as being replicated rapidly. This can be helpful for sharing information for therapy interventions, for example a series of five-minute exercises. The flash cards could be tailored and used as the basis for a short personalised video to support therapy aims and goals. They can also be downloaded as PDFs. This means if a video is recorded and shared with an individual, the corresponding set of cards can be sent using one of the secure methods outlined in Section 2 and makes for a fully digital therapy programme that the individual can follow at home. They can be kept as sets of exercises and build a bank of resources over time, migrating to develop digital resources for areas of therapy such as phonology, where these take time and patience but are highly reusable once created and can be saved and shared with multiple individuals or settings.

Examples of where to find online flash cards and how to create and use them can be found in the resources section.

GREEN SCREEN DREAM

Ever wondered how you could make magic happen on screen? Wonder no longer and prepare to add a little magic into your digital toolkit and your sessions by incorporating green screens into therapy. This technique works really well with children and young people of all ages and can be easily adapted to fit their special interests, introduce a topic or character or just about anything else you can think of.

It could be used very effectively in nursery, for example using particular characters that are known for having bags, as a whole class resource for sensory stories to establish engagement, deliver language groups or early phonics. The same resource could be used for 1:1 sessions in language, phonics, social skills, but also preparation and transition for key points such as new class, teacher introduction, school transitions, personal life event changes such as new babies, house moves, etc. could also make use of this. This particular example has been adapted from a version that was originally created as part of a college transition. For the purpose of the permissions no images or characters that require licensing used in the images. If you wish to use to specific characters as part of special interests or topics make sure you are not breaching and licensing or permissions that may be associated with them.

HOW TO ... CREATE A PERSONALISED GREEN SCREEN RECORDING!

You will need:

- A large piece of green paper or felt tacked to the wall behind where you sit at your laptop. This will also need a pocket for the visuals you are going to pull out (in the example video, it is Dora's backpack). When using Teams, images will need to be saved as a .PNG, .JPG or .BMP file, so remember to change the file type before saving.

- Visuals or objects of whatever you want to pull from the backpack, satchel, cupboard, etc. need to be printed or small enough to place in the pocket.
- A Zoom account or MS Teams account and a laptop/computer. This is important particularly for Zoom, as without an account and having the app downloaded you will have reduced functionality and changing background is one of these!

STEPS 1 and 2

1. Begin a Zoom or MS Teams call, but with yourself as the only participant (you can do this by sending yourself an invite!).
2. Once in the call, press 'share screen' in Zoom in the bar along the bottom of the screen or the icon in Teams.

STEP 3

3. In MS Teams, either select 'Background Filters' when setting up camera and audio *or* click the three dots and select 'Background Settings'.

- To use the new picture for the background, select 'Add New' and then select the relevant file to upload from your computer. Make sure when you save the picture it's a .JPG, .PNG or .BMP file.
- In Zoom, select 'Advanced'.
- Select 'PowerPoint as virtual background' and press 'Share'. This will bring up your folders. Locate the chosen PowerPoint and select as the virtual background choice.
- Make sure you don't have this PowerPoint open on your laptop already, as it won't open as a background if it is 'in use' already.

STEP 4

4. You are now 'in' the PowerPoint. Position yourself so when you reach into the pocket on the green screen, you are reaching into the bag on the screen.

STEPS 5 and 6

5. Once you are happy with the positioning, you can press 'record' next to 'share screen' and begin your video!
6. When you are finished, stop recording and the link will be sent to your email address registered for you to edit, if you wish, or simply download and share or play! (See Figure 39.1.)

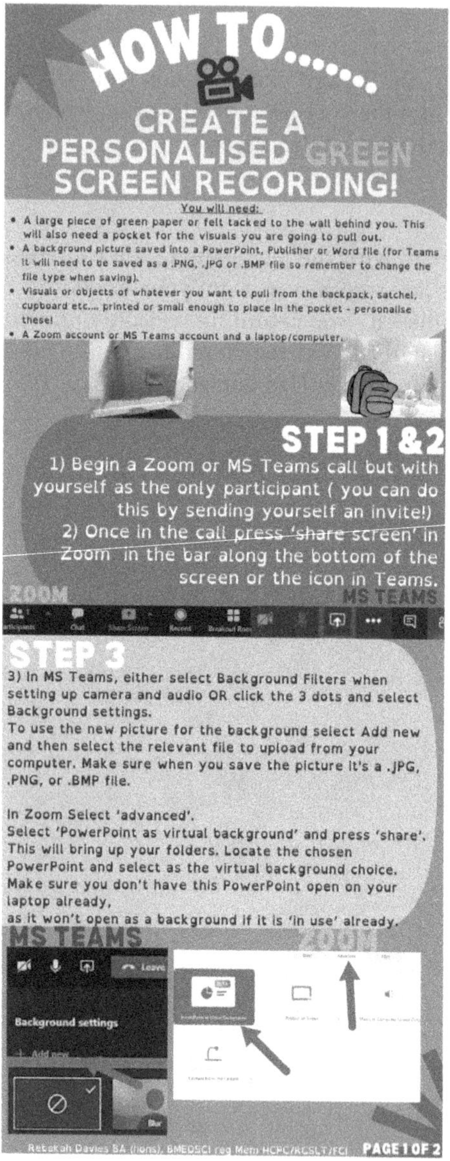

Figure 39.1 How to …

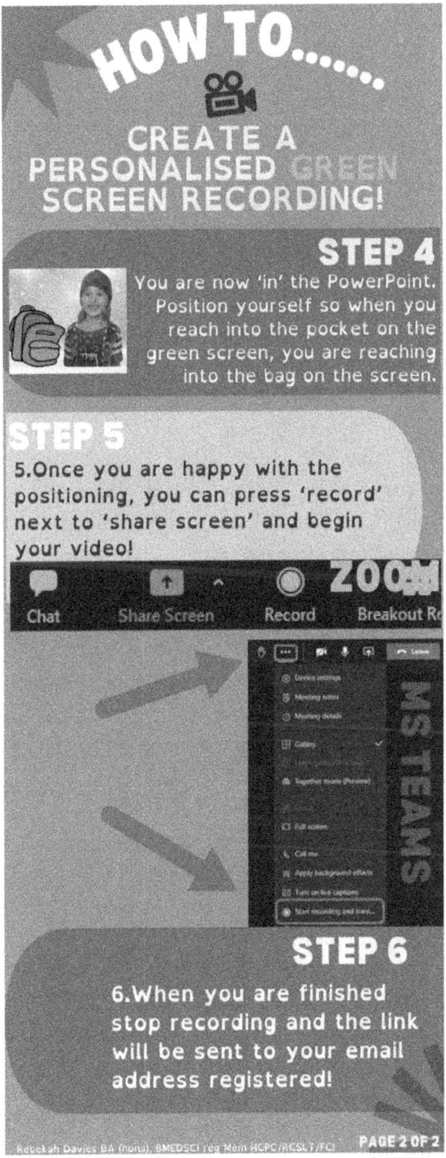

Figure 39.1 How to ... (continued)

CENTRE OF THE CAREVERSE: TAILORING PLANS

The people we care for, whether the terminology we use in our settings to refer to them is patient, service user, client, student, learner or pupil, are at the centre of any interventions we plan. We are person-centred.

It's sometimes easy to forget this when there's so much else going on to manage: time, date, delivery method, therapy model, resources to make, MDT meetings to attend, reports to write, referrals to make, where's the person?

Creating personalised care plans not only keep the person at the heart of the planning but they are documents that can be invaluable in sharing information quickly and easily with different professionals for different reasons at different times, and the best bit? The person themselves can be involved in developing and updating these. It allows someone to have real engagement in their own healthcare as well as providing a snap shot into their healthcare story.

Many therapists are familiar with care plans, whether this is from an adult perspective in a residential home setting or paediatric perspective and the pen portraits that are often produced for children receiving additional Special Educational Need and Disability (SEND) support across primary and into secondary and Key Stage 3, depending on the setting.

From a therapeutic perspective, having a one-page, person-centred care plan is useful. It should be kept as part of the person's profile that can provide key information such as,

- Photo, if possible, for identification (particularly useful for identification during remote consultations).

DOI: 10.4324/9781003269724-44

- Medications.
- Recent surgery or pending procedures.
- Emergency details.
- Key conditions or contraindications.
- Therapy objectives.
- Preferred methods of engagement (email, SMS, video, letter, etc.) that can be updated regularly. This should ideally be checked at each session to ensure the care being delivered is person-centred and takes into account the person's preferences and choices.

These documents can be quickly and easily produced and shared electronically via secure email or approved SMS with relevant professionals ensuring that the care and interventions you are providing are known to other professionals and can be added to the records if using differing systems. These can be particularly useful for quickly sharing your input, recapping therapy goals, including as a visual addition to a written report and sharing with the person to ensure they are happy with it and can inform if there are any changes that they would like to make or information to add.

There are numerous methods to produce, but one tool I particularly have found a lot of uses for and keep finding them is Canva!

This online creativity tool was initially intended to design great social media posts to make them engaging and easily editable. One of the best features about this online software is it has lots of free to use templates.

The tool is free access with the option of a premium account to unlock everything which new users get a free trial for and is highly recommended.

The templates I use the most are the infographics. These are long, thin visuals (think an A4 sheet cut lengthways). I've used these for organisation and operational planning through to infographics produced for national guidelines.

Canva allows the user to use all the accessibility knowledge gained in Chapter 34 about creating accessible documents using Microsoft tools and apply it to other digital tools to provide wider opportunities and options for engagement.

From selecting dyslexia-friendly fonts, tracking and colour, to embedding videos with sign language or Makaton to accompany a presentation, all of these can be added into documents within this tool.

Another feature I really like is the collaboration element, and again personalising an experience. For those familiar with creating PowerPoint presentations, many of the features are the same with the bonus of tenplates being there as inspiration if you are struggling for ideas to get you started. Using Canva is no scarier than PowerPoint, plus you can share a link and edit the document with other people in tandem in real time!

From a therapy perspective this strategy could be used for informal assessments, simple turn-taking or language games that can be tailored to special interests by downloading images from the web or uploading from your device files. Examples might include,

- Dress the character – (choose a favourite animal, cartoon character or person) and add a range of accessories in different sizes and colours for discrimination purposes.
- Create a scene – use a template picture and add people, objects, etc. and create a scenario or story as part of narrative exercises.
- Comic book story – great for emotions exploring and social skills, moral questions – 'what would you do if?', 'what do you think this character should do?' You can choose characters from images available, upload photos or find suitable images online to add to your bank of available images. Easily add new frames of pages to the document to extend the story, then present the document as an animation, presentation or share as a file and add it to their record as a recording of session goals and outcomes success.
- Preposition activities – monster prepositions have always been a favourite and this is a step up from me laminating odd-shaped, brightly coloured creatures stuck to a piece

of card with hook and loop tape! As Canva automatically stores all your designs online (you don't even need to save them, although you can, just for additional peace of mind), so you can mix and match resources once you've made them to extend the options you have (e.g. use the backgrounds from create a scene and introduce a monster or two for prepositions). You can easily revisit favourite games you've created with a particular individual as everything is in one place. You can even create folders if you want to assign to specific people or places, e.g. all St Aurora's school activities in one folder and Lily Lane in another.

- Empower me – an activity I prepared for a group of young people with learning difficulties was to use the idea of a digital version of a communication board. The boards could be personalised to allow individuals to share their opinions, ideas, wants and needs during a co-design session for a digital design project. The learners preferred different types of communication expression and so they were created to allow one learner to type, one to use single words/phrases and another to use images or icons to express their ideas.

- I used key phrases, yes, no, maybe and the option of emoticons to point to for the learner who preferred short phrases with some blank 'Post-Its' for dynamic additions, too. For others who were really familiar with using pictures and symbols to communicate, I selected or uploaded relevant images and added them to their board to move about during the session in response to questions. All of these were made available as Canva allowed me to copy the document, make adjustments and allow each learner their own tool to engage and interact during the session. These could also be saved for the next session and shared stored in their electronic records by staff working with them as part of their therapy within their educational settings.

See the resources section for an example of a personalised care plan, activities and tools using Canva.

41

TEAM OF 1! CREATING PERSONALISED VIDEO CONTENT TO SUPPORT THERAPY

Ever found yourself talking to, well, yourself? Well if you haven't before you absolutely will if you go ahead and create personalised video content. Whether you are creating a fantasy version with a Green Screen (Chapter 39) or you are creating a bespoke video to accompany a series of new exercises…panic not! We are not about to set up a new social media site for speech and language therapists where you'll be required to bake a Bolognese whilst salsa dancing and doing a uvular trill (although now I'm thinking this sounds like a challenge, but in the name of clinical safety, step away from the pasta shells!).

Instead of dancing up a storm, you can do something much more straightforward and something you've probably done a lot without thinking about, send a video link. Except this time, the only recipient will be you!

This might seem slightly strange, but it's just so you can access the link, join the meeting and record and receive the link back from the content you've recorded.

So, now you know what on earth talking to yourself might be useful for, what is the content of these solo performances?

One area that works really well in video format is sharing information. Increasingly consent forms part of what we do when working digitally, especially informed consent.

We looked earlier at assumed consent for participating in video consultations, assumed on the basis that if someone accepts a link they are happy to continue with the consultation, but maybe you want to ensure someone has had all the

DOI: 10.4324/9781003269724-45

options of their care shared with them, that they understand the implications and rules of group participation or that they agree to doing their therapy regularly.

More often than not, this has been a one-page document shared early on in therapy on a printed piece of paper or, with changing landscapes, these are turned into PDF formats and shared as attached to an email or SMS (securely, of course), but now it can be a spoken, visual, living document! The video in this instance could be a personalised version of the consent form, addressing an individual directly. A great strategy for gaining the attention of individuals, or anyone who can find it hard to attend to general information and you need to grab the attention of for important information!

Other purposes of a personalised video could be,

- Specific therapy exercises – from Lax Vox to Masako or even a short video of sequencing tasks for making a cup of tea for an aphasia patient, to support functional memory following stroke.
- To set therapy goals and objectives.
- To record a reading passage for an individual to play back and practice with.
- Breathing exercises to regulate breathing.
- Phonology activities for older children to follow more complex tasks independently.
- Setting secret missions or tasks for teens or young adults.

To share it, depending on size of the file, it can be attached electronically to communications to be shared and added to electronic health records, or the link generated by recording can be added directly within an email or SMS, or you can create a webpage such as a SharePoint site to host the link on and then send a link to this if the file is larger than average. If this is the case you will usually get a prompt from the mail server to suggest sending by an alternate means.

Remember where possible to create a download version and then save it on your cloud drive in a folder, just in case.

SO, WHAT ELSE MIGHT IT BE USEFUL FOR?

- Consent – see above.
- Transition preparation for individuals or groups to or from education settings.
- Introductions for new professionals supporting a person.
- Therapy exercises – introduction of a new one, modelling current or ongoing ones (a great tool to ensure that exercises, especially voice-specific, are being modelled properly – you are a therapist in a pocket and can be carried wherever they go, home or away).
- Goal setting – again, really specific and clear, broken down for each goal that can be revisited for reference as many times as needed.
- See resources for PDF of how to create a personalised video.

42

SAY AHHH: GETTING THE
BEST INTRA-ORAL IMAGES

Fancy taking a tons-elfie? I couldn't resist, but, it's actually not beyond the realms of the impossible that taking a selfie of tonsils, tongue and teeth are skills that certain clinical groups can benefit from!

Diagnosing disorders of swallow, voice and phonology, as well as investigating palate and checking cranial nerves all require familiarity with and clear vision of the oral cavity. These assessments are more than laryngeal palpation, physically assessing adequate elevation and excursion of the larynx, the simple fact is mouth care really does matter and being able to see the interior of an oral cavity can tell us a lot about an individual's current health as well as any barrier to oral intake, including masticatory factors as well as general hygiene and hydration.

So, how can we use technology to maximise our visuals during virtuals? As with many aspects of virtual consults and as any self-respecting oral selfie-er will advise, it's all about the lighting (and spoons!).

WHAT YOU'LL NEED

- A mobile device with a front-facing, flash-enabled camera.
- Separate pen torch.
- Clip-on selfie ring.
- Two metal dessert spoons (adult) for a child. Depending on size of oral cavity, teaspoons may work, especially with a smaller mouth!
- An extra pair of hands is easiest, so one person can take the photo and one can use the spoons to maximise the best angle of the oral cavity where possible.

DOI: 10.4324/9781003269724-46

These are methods of providing images to support both clinical decision making and inform therapy aims and objectives. They are intended to be an additional tool, utilising digital pathways to enhance safety and reduce the risk of infection for both patient and clinician. They may be useful in a variety of contexts in both adult and paediatric settings. The following examples are suggestions of how images could be used within a range of scenarios.

- Individuals undergoing radiotherapy to reduce their in-person appointments and minimise infection risk.
- To reduce episodes of aerosol-generating procedures, as has been the case throughout the Covid-19 pandemic and beyond.
- View dentition and any structural impact on phonology.
- As part of cranial nerve assessment – including any weakness or paralysis.
- Any palatal abnormalities that may be impacting speech or feeding.
- Allow clinicians the ability to offer mouth care advice to carers around increasing oral comfort and secretion management of an individual who may otherwise have been admitted for a swallow-related referral. Quality of life may be improved and admission may be prevented.
- Visual baseline for treatment when and if appropriate and if agreed by the individual. An example of such may be jaw opening where trismus from the effects of radiotherapy has been impacted. Some individuals respond effectively to visual markers and they can be a way of tracking their therapy goals and journey as it can be hard to remember progress, especially when we measure it in millimetres and so often have only a written report to reflect on.

TAKING THE IMAGE

This may depend slightly on what information you, as the clinician, are intending to achieve or the individual is aiming to share. It may be helpful to have scripts of information ready to share depending on what you would like to receive on an image.

EXAMPLE 1

Advice that can be adapted and shared.

SIMPLE ORAL CAVITY IMAGE – STRAIGHT ON

- Ensure you are against a white or light background where possible.
- Gently place a spoon convex (rounded) side facing into the side of each cheek and gently hold the spoon handles apart.
- Hold your mouth as wide open as you can and say, 'Ahhh'.
- Ask someone to take a close-up photograph that includes your whole mouth.

EXAMPLE 2

HARD AND SOFT PALATE VIEW

- Ensure you are against a white or light background where possible.
- Gently place a spoon convex (rounded) side facing into the side of each cheek and gently hold the spoon handles apart.
- Open your mouth wide and lift your chin as much as you can. Make sure the person taking the photograph can see all the palate.
- Hold the camera so that it's as close to 90° as possible to the biting surface of your top teeth.

EXAMPLE 3

TONGUE

Useful for glossectomy or partial glossectomy and management.

- Ensure you are against a white or light background where possible.
- Gently place a spoon convex (rounded) side facing into the side of each cheek and gently hold the spoon handles apart.

Figure 42.1 Intra-oral images with spoons

LEFT SIDE

- Bite down naturally with your back teeth touching.
- Use a spoon to pull back your cheek and lips to show all your back teeth on the LEFT.
- If it uncomfortable at any time, remove the spoons, reposition and try again.
  WHY IS THIS ANGLE USEFUL ?
- It's important to check the whole mouth wherever possible and look for any potential causes of discomfort or problems that might impact eating and drinking.

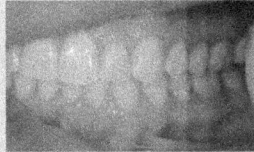

UPPER PALATE

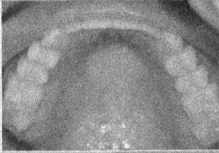

- Open your mouth wide and lift your chin as much as you can.
- Hold the camera so that it's as level as possible to the biting surface of your top teeth.
- Make sure you can see as much of the palate as possible- you could take two images one for soft and one for hard with head tilted to slightly different angles.
  WHY IS THIS ANGLE USEFUL?
- This angle can give an indication of oral hygiene, changes or hydration, e.g. if dried secretions are present on the hard and soft palate or the back of the mouth (known as the pharyngeal wall)

LOWER PALATE

- Open your mouth wide and tilt your chin downwards towards your chest.
- Hold the camera so that it's as perpendicular as possible to the biting surfaces of your bottom teeth.
- Make sure all your teeth are showing!
  WHY IS THIS ANGLE USEFUL?
- **This view is useful for reviewing the lower palate and any concerns or changes that may need further investigation .**
- **It's also great to assess and monitor recovery after tongue surgery (partial or full glossectomy)**

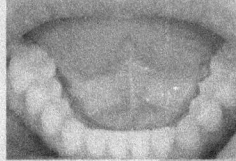

Rebekah Davies
HPEC and RCSLT registered Speech and Language Therapist
UHCT Member
@RemotelyPossibs

Figure 42.1 Intra-oral images with spoons (continued)

- Open your mouth wide and tilt your chin downwards towards your chest.
- Hold the camera so that it's as perpendicular as possible to the biting surfaces of your bottom teeth.
- Ask someone you feel comfortable with to take the four images,
  1. From the centre natural position.
  2. To the right.
  3. To the left.
  4. Tongue between teeth (modified dependent on goals).
- Do not over stretch so that it is uncomfortable (see Figure 42.1).

GETTING ATTACHED: SHARING, RECEIVING AND SAVING ATTACHMENTS SAFELY

Attachments on emails and SMS are part of our daily routine, 'click here to download', 'follow this link' or 'see attachment' are all familiar phrases in our daily digital lives, but what are the purposes of needing to do this in a clinical setting, how does it differ? In Section 2 we learned the significance of secure emails and how to create instances of secure email chains for NHS Mail users but, more generally, how do we send, receive and store attachments safely?

Firstly, establishing a purpose for attachments is important. They can range from a clinician sending out digital appointment letters, electronic feedback forms or individualised therapy programs to an individual sharing images, reports from external agencies or anecdotal information from a family member. All examples may have patient-identifiable information, which has the potential to risk breaching confidentiality and impact patient safety, whether shared via email or approved SMS provider.

As per the guidance in Section 2, sharing information should only be done as part of a secure email chain or with another secure and trusted email address. Your organisation will be able to provide you with a list of email suffixes that are approved as 'safe' and may include government agencies, the defence sector and other healthcare organisations.

Once the information is received, the most important thing is that this is transferred as quickly as possible to the relevant individual's record. The information may not be time-sensitive but, the longer it is available on a server, the more risk there is of someone accessing it intentionally or unintentionally. Whenever you are handling patient-identifiable information think, 'if this was my/my family's information, who would I want to see it?'

To safely open and store an attachment you have received from a trusted source,

1. Either copy the information if it is in the body of an email or SMS and simply copy and paste into the person's record. Alternatively, if the information requires downloading first, download to a trusted device. I always do this onto the desktop so I can transfer quickly and easily and then delete the file with minimum effort.
2. From the desktop, upload into the relevant folder, page or file within the electronic record, ensuring it is clearly labelled and dated.
3. Once the attachment has been uploaded and any additional information relevant to the attachment recorded in the record, delete the file made on the desktop and delete the email in order to ensure confidentiality and security.

ATTACHMENTS FROM A NON-SECURE SOURCE

Phishing emails are increasingly common and sophisticated in their content. Cyber criminals are becoming more adept at infiltrating networks and analysing the content of organisational emails in order to replicate them and use them to obtain information or data by illegal means. They can appear to be extremely convincing and even appear to be from within your own organisation or an arm of it, such as informing you that a download of software is due to upgrade your device and you must open an attachment immediately to avoid action which may be anything from not having access to emails through to disciplinary measures for non-compliance.

Identifying a phishing email and attachment can be difficult, but if you are tuned in and alert it's not impossible and will save you and your colleagues not only time but may protect those in our care also.

The National Cyber Security Centre (NCSC) has a wealth of advice in identifying and reporting suspicious emails, text messages or phone calls.

The email or message may be from an email address that doesn't look in a format you may expect, for example it may have a lot of numbers rather than someone's name.

There may be grammatical or spelling errors – (warning, deliberate spelling mistake alert) – it is unlikely that NHS Digital, for example, would alert you to an 'imminent network failure' or inform you that 'your account will be suspended unless you open the attachment and return the requested information immediately'.

These are subtle devices used to instil fear and threaten. There are ways to check whether they are genuine without opening them and are procedures you can follow to ensure as few people as possible are disrupted.

- Firstly, don't open any emails or messages you think may be suspicious. They may open a type of device called malware that collects information from your device and any networks you are connected to. This may include patient data. It can make your device stop working properly and corrupt existing information and files you may have stored.
- Forward them to your information governance department or follow your organisational policies for phishing emails or messages. They may request they are reported to the National Cyber Security Centre using report@phishing.gov.uk.
- Be vigilant. Advise your colleagues what to look out for. Cyber criminals will use 'campaigns' linked to your organisation's work to make them look convincing to you. If you're not expecting an update, chances are there isn't one due to happen!
- If you are in any doubt, check with your information governance leads who will be able to advise further.

44

QR-LITY: UTILISING QR CODES IN THERAPY AND EVALUATION

Quick Response or QR codes were briefly discussed in Section 2, Chapter 10 – The Big Click On. A camera-friendly barcode that we can use for everything from accessing evaluation forms to directing to personalised interventions or signposting to specific videos online. They are capable of holding a lot of data in a very small area and each is unique. I described them previously as being like a fingerprint due to each one being completely unique. QR codes are a visual representation of a digital location, a little bit like giving a document or webpage a virtual address. They can be linked directly to a website as we are most familiar with so, for example, we might create a code that is linked to our organisation's website and a further one that directs visitors to a specific page within the website to find out more about therapy.

QR codes can be used for other types of information, too.

EVALUATION

Surveys, questionnaires or assessments are a great use of this digital tool in therapy. Once the code is created it can be used over and over again as a fixed point on a website or webpage, or it could be copy and pasted onto letters and into SMS or emails.

The assessments, questionnaires or subjective scales themselves may be existing tools that are standardised and widely accepted or may be local versions that are used with a specific organisation. They may have been purchased as digital versions or adapted into digital versions using simple tools such as Microsoft Forms, Survey Monkey, Qualtrics, Google or Jot Form (but there are others).

166

DOI: 10.4324/9781003269724-48

Evaluation is a powerful tool of any service and particularly so for digital pathways. Quality data is needed in order to learn, develop and iteratively innovate pathways in order that we provide the best care to fit the needs of the individuals in the way that they are choosing to engage and receive care. The more data we have, the more we can understand where improvements need to be made, where efficiencies should be focussed and how we can best meet the evolving needs of those we care for. If we have poor quality data inputted, we can't expect quality data to be the output. In other words, you can't polish mud and expect diamonds!

WHERE AND WHEN?

QR codes have a place in both individual and group therapy and can be a quick and easy way of directing to information for a variety of purposes depending on the session content, participants and aims. It may be that they are used,

- Before the session to collate subjective perceptions or beliefs about therapy and goals.
- During 1:1 sessions or group workshops for collating and sharing ideas.
- Completing polls and engaging in collaborative activities.
- Post-feedback and quality improvement forms, signposting for ongoing therapy activities, online activities and resources that are updated after each session.

QR CODES – THEY'RE NOT JUST FOR ONLINE, THEY'RE FOR REAL LIFE!

Digital tools aren't just for online only, but can turn the ordinary into extraordinary. making that in-person session that little bit more engaging and challenging to support those all-important therapy objectives.

Older children and young adults particularly may engage well with activities using their own familiar mobile devices in conjunction with QR codes, although confident KS1 and 2 children with appropriate equipment at school could engage equally as competently in small groups or teams if devices aren't available for one each.

Activities that it may be possible to set up using QR codes include a treasure or scavenger hunt, murder mystery or escape room-type activity, plus other similar activities such as a straightforward quiz where the QR code provides an answer or clue.

The QR codes are merely the vehicle for improving social skills by encouraging working collaboratively, problem solving, building independence, through to increasing navigation and direction skills of a new building or area.

This method of using digital tools as part of a blended or hybrid toolkit could be used, for example, to support transition to a new setting, using the QR codes to mark out different destinations with clues to solve that lead to the next.

These hopefully will generate some more 'QR-lity' ideas of how QR codes could be utilised in your therapy directly or indirectly. You may be already using them creatively in your work, feel free to share your tips and ideas using #remotelyresources and tagging @RemotelyPossib1.

Section 4

A REMOTELY POSSIBLE FUTURE

45

LONG-TERM PLANNING: DEVELOPING DIGITAL SPEECH AND LANGUAGE THERAPY SERVICES

Planning for the long term can be easier said than done when we don't know what we are planning for, and because it can feel like managing an entirely different service if you suddenly think about it as a digital service if it isn't one currently. It's hard to try and plan for the future when tomorrow might still be an unknown!

For this reason it may be easier to segment what the future may hold by building the foundations and working towards a solid digital service than trying to throw everything at it and it collapsing because no one knew about it, there was no training and the technology you were using wasn't built to accommodate what you were aiming for, and that's before you introduce the public!

These are a few considerations that may help build digital into the future of SLT services. They are not exhaustive, and your local health informatics teams will be happy to support you with transformation projects, talking to your teams and understanding the challenges you are experiencing that may be creating any barriers to introducing digital into your services.

1. *Too many cooks* … It's great if you have enthusiastic team members, but having one person that can coordinate your digital work can be much more helpful than it being split by several who aren't as committed as one individual who really wants to explore this area of their development.

2. Look at digital health or 'clinical informatics' as a specialism in the same way that all other elements of the profession are. It may help the team member to start to build a profile as a digital lead within the team and the wider organisation (that's how I started). If the role is core to the team, the individual could have targets built into their CPD and Personal Development Review (PDR) so they are developing their own career as well as enhancing the aims of the service. Consider this individual being the one to represent the service in digital meetings from a directorate perspective and beyond.

3. It's important to understand the organisation's digital strategy and digital agenda and where your service fits within that. Ask yourself and those within health informatics (CIO, CCIO, for example).

- How can you be involved?
- Where are you or your service on that journey already?
- How receptive are your service/team, as much of the work is change management and winning hearts and minds as it is about implementing new technology.
- Consider the fact that as humans we are not always comfortable with change, and because of this it's important to include those around us in new decisions and information to ensure they are aware of the rationale and reason behind why these changes are happening.
- Remember – digital isn't a secret that should happen behind closed doors. Ensuring transparency means that everyone can be on the same page and work towards the same clear objectives. Joined-up care is better care and data saves lives! Where transformation happens these outcomes can be more efficiently achieved with digital an enabler for this across all specialities.

4. Do you know who to approach for help? Familiarise yourself with the roles of digital and the hierarchy within your organisation (see Chapter 46).

5. Consider which parts of the service you could digitise. This may be making better use of information flows in the EPR, using new parts of the video consultation software to enhance consultations, such as feedback surveys, introducing self-management tools to reduce waiting time for people waiting for triage that may be able to resolve the problem they are experiencing with remote guidance and completing an online diary that is uploaded to their electronic record. Start simple and see and measure the impact. This will reassure the team that digital can be useful and supportive of services as well as hopefully give them the confidence to approach the next step in adding further digital processes into the service.

6. Never be afraid to ask for help. You are not alone. The success of a whole organisation is not based on the actions of one service, it is based on the whole of an organisation acting as one service so that everything works together, is streamlined and benefits those that are being cared for as much as those doing the caring.

46

HEALTH INFORMATICS AND BEYOND: ACRONYMS AND ASKING FOR HELP

I previously mentioned being familiar with your local Health Informatics team, but who are the key stakeholders that make decisions?

As I'm familiar with the NHS titles these are the ones I will use, but there may be slightly different variations even within the NHS depending on the size of trust and even more variation outside of this.

From my perspective, the main stakeholders that an SLT service is likely to come across within their organisation are CIO, CCIO, CNIO, CAHPIO, DCSO, EPR lead. It may look at first sight like the first half of the alphabet thrown in the air and reformed in various ways, but what do all these acronyms mean?

CIO: Chief Information Officer – this is the main person and the title usually sits with the head of director of informatics. The role may also be known as CDIO or Chief Digital Officer, it may also be assigned a director-level acronym. This role is significant. They are budget holders, directors, decision makers and highly influential. They are forward thinkers who see opportunity everywhere and interoperability (even the very word) is their weakness!

CCIO: Chief Clinical Information Officer – this role can be a clinician from any clinical background aligned to the health informatics department who works in close alignment with the CIO and other roles. Some are also DSCO-accredited but are dependent on the individual. However, historically (although

DOI: 10.4324/9781003269724-51

no one really understands why) it is often assumed it has to be a consultant-grade medical doctor that takes on this role. This is not hugely accurate, and the Faculty of Clinical Informatics have recently developed a job description for CCIOs to support standardising as it has become political in recent times around clinicians potentially having been assigned roles when the stipulations following the Wachter and Topol reviews outlined that every medium-sized NHS organisation should have at least four CCIOs, most have one and whilst some still don't have an assigned role this is increasingly rare, as informatics cements itself within clinical professions. Nationally we have a CCIO (Chief Clinical Information Officer) with a national CNIO (Chief Nursing Information Officer) – the informatics lead for nurses, separate to the Chief Nurse. As with the CCIO, they work alongside the informatics team, usually on nursing transformations, although they do get involved with wider projects and support colleagues wherever their skill mix is required. NHSX now known as the Transformation Directorate has been one of the arms of the national bodies of the NHS and is a collaboration of NHS England and Improvement and Department of Health and Social Care, but will be part of a wider merge with NHS England and Improvement alongside NHS Digital and Health Education England to streamline digital transformation across the NHS.

CAHPIO: Chief Allied Health Profession Information Officer – yes, it's a mouthful, but sadly these roles are few and far between and we are typically represented by the CNIOs or CCIOs, which don't accurately reflect our AHP backgrounds or experiences. This is one of the reasons the role of the CCIO is being challenged so that more professions who are eligible to apply, albeit except they aren't GMC registered, can undertake the roles. AHPs do not have a national CAHPIO, unlike CCIOs and CNIOs, Natasha Phillips nationally is supposed to represent AHPs as well as nurses, but this is being disputed for the reasons outlined above, as we are quite different to nurses and digital AHPs feel we are not represented effectively. The national AHP lead is aware of the digital agenda and it is covered by AHPs into Action, but many AHPs feel strongly this isn't sufficient in terms of representation in the digital sphere and feel an AHPIO is warranted.

EPR lead: Electronic Patient Record lead – this role may be titled several things depending on the organisation, but is typically aligned to the management of the electronic health record and anything from a clinical system perspective that needs to connect with it. This individual will have a significant role in the orgsanisation and in some organisations may deputise for the CIO.

D/CSO: Digital Clinical Safety Officer – responsible for ensuring new technology or digital processes such as transferring paper-based processes to a digital format, introducing a new app, voice recognition software or video consultation platform. This would all go through a hazard workshop with the relevant stakeholders, i.e. the people using the technology or impacted by the deployment and a full report written up to highlight any risks and a mitigation plan.

DIGITAL ENHANCEMENTS OF PRACTICE: DEVELOPING YOUR DIGITAL ASSETS

Weaving digital into how you enhance practice is relatively easy, as I could pretty much guarantee you've searched something on the internet today? It might not have been CPD-related, but applying the same methods to the scenario you are researching or have set your CPD aims around is one method of using digital tools to enhance your learning.

There are a huge amount of free resources available on the internet and I've shared references to some in other sections, such as the accessibility tools and learning Microsoft provides free of charge.

Other organisations provide digital skills and digital support to enhance practice, whether it be an online resource you are studying remotely as a distance-learning module, YouTube or TikTok video or a course specific to your objectives, there is something to cover most needs, be it clinical, digital or both.

At present there is no standardised pathway for clinicians to be skilled in delivering video consultations. I am aware that there are several organisations that offer role play training to enhance confidence of delivering remote consultations, and there are instances of NHS England and Improvement piloting some solutions to understand if they have measurable impact for their clinicians and on the service outcomes (engagement, clinical decision making, confidence in using digital tools etc.).

There are also some organisations who have developed their own training modules specific to the virtual consultation platforms they are using.

DOI: 10.4324/9781003269724-52

The reality is, for the public, depending on the organisation they are receiving healthcare from the virtual input they are offered depends on whether the clinician they are seeing has had any training to deliver virtual care beyond 'press here'.

This is one element of CPD that has become significant in my current role and I have been looking at existing pathways to understand what needs to be available in order to ensure virtual consultations are delivered by competent and confident clinicians to not only ensure better outcomes for the individual receiving the care, but to reduce any potential health inequalities that may arise from not having received any training.

Of course this is only one area of CPD that a clinician may need to undertake and digital could be used to deliver experiences that, until now, haven't been options due to geographical boundaries. For example, a student could participate in a virtual placement in Scotland despite being at home in Cornwall, thereby being exposed to different clinical experiences and demographics whereby broadening their awareness and understanding as a new clinician. It also allows for expert input from clinicians seeking peer support from those nationally or in extreme circumstances seeking expertise globally on the same call, in the same MDT for the benefit of the same individual. Previously this may have been all through letter or email, at best slowing down outcomes and decision making for treatment.

Digital can help us do more, do better and do it differently. Think outside the box, what do you want to experience and achieve in your CPD? Could you ask for input from a colleague in America, could you observe an SLT in Ireland or are you interested in a piece of research happening in Spain? Digital has no borders and we can use that to our benefit. Yes, explore what is familiar and known, but our options are infinitely increased by having digital tools to support us in our research, our career progressions and enhancing our practice.

BURN BABY BURN: MANAGING SCREEN BURNOUT

Do you remember at the start of lockdown in 2020, all of those Zoom parties, the online pub quizzes everyone did with family and friends? They were amazing, and they served a great purpose – to help everyone feel connected, but then they just fizzled out. As more of our work went online, the less time we wanted to speak with our friends online, the screen fatigue was more and more evident.

I remember speaking to a friend who was a receptionist at one point in her life. She told me she hated speaking to people on the phone in her personal time, because that's all she did in her work day. Perhaps a case of too much of a good thing where we do one thing to excess.

If this is what we are navigating, how do we maintain that balance?

Screen burnout or the fatigue described previously is a very real thing. Did you know that it was reported by the Stanford Virtual Human Interaction Lab (2021) that continuous screen meetings actually add to fatigue,decreased mobility and and increased cognitive load! Whilst MIND (2022)highlights that whilst burnout doesn't refer to a diagnosis itself, it is instead indicative of a collection of symptoms. If you are experiencing burnout you may feel completely exhausted, have little motivation for your job, feel irritable, or anxious and you may see a dip in your work performance. Some people also experience physical symptoms like headaches or stomach aches, or have trouble sleeping.

Whilst this is a developing area of research there are emerging studies about the effects of screen fatigue, including recent studies by Bailensen (2021). He outlines several suggestions for reducing screen fatigue when working for extended periods of time and recognises the differences this way of working has on our psychological selves, including seeing yourself on screen multiple times a day.

It's important to recognise the warning signs of burnout so that we are able to mitigate and minimise before it spirals out of control and stress levels increase disproportionately to the tasks at hand.

There are simple steps we can all take to prevent an attack of burnout and protect ourselves from the associated fatigue that can be exhausting at best and crippling at worst.

MAKE SURE YOU TAKE YOUR ANNUAL LEAVE

A lot of people haven't taken as much holiday from work as they normally might recently due to changes in travel, cancellations in planned trips and caring for families or loved ones at home. However, just because we aren't leaving the country doesn't mean we can't leave the keyboard!

Taking time off is just as important even if you are having a day at home, pottering in the allotment, having a day of retail therapy, spa day or meeting with friends. Whatever you do, even if it's a day catching up on box sets eating chocolate, it gives you an opportunity to relax and recharge.

GET ENOUGH SLEEP

It sounds so obvious and fundamental, but many of us don't get good sleep. The sort of sleep that you wake up feeling that you've actually been to sleep instead of tossing and turning most of the night. If you struggle to get to sleep a digital detox in the bedroom can help switch off...literally. Leaving phone chargers downstairs so you have to charge your device away from where you sleep can help some individuals who are using tech tools throughout the day as a strategy to shut down.

Blue or white light can prevent the brain switching off or powering down. It's the way in which our body creates melatonin to support sleep and the lights of phones and laptops actually prevent this from happening. As someone who doesn't make much naturally, I need all the help I can get, so turning off screens can be an easy way to help your brain begin the switch off. If you really can't manage without your phone or your relaxing activity is on it, such as reading on your reading app, try altering the lighting, size of font and colour of the background to reduce glare and soften the lighting and signals received by your brain. Most phones have a night mode and you can set night mode using the accessibility settings on Windows devices, too (see Chapter 34).

Trying other relaxing activities before you go to bed at night can help, too. See a list of suggestions in Chapter 49 – How's Your Head?.

TRY TO FINISH WORK ON TIME

Without the commute and with the pressures of home-schooling, it's easier to work late into the evening to try and get everything done. We have all worked over our hours over the last few months, but doing this regularly can impact our overall wellbeing as we compensate in other areas of our lives as work begins to infringe on our personal lives.

It's now possible to book in a 'virtual commute' using Microsoft Teams. A chance to a acknowledge the time between leaving work and arriving home, where to-do lists are written, the following day is planned and pencilled in and you can prepare to shut down and begin your evening. It might not be a tool that works for everyone, but it could be worth trying out to see if it fits with your schedule and activities to help plan and declutter your brain from a day at the desk. (See online resources for virtual commutes.)

SCHEDULE IN TIME FOR FUN!

Make time for the things you enjoy doing. From bubble baths to walking the dog, a phone call with friends or a long-forgotten craft you have been meaning to try your hand at. Set time aside for you on a regular basis. You might prefer small chunks throughout the week or one longer chunk for a whole afternoon. Whatever works for you, having something non-work related to look forward to can really help, and with the ability to work flexibly, managing a little 'me' time is perhaps a little less like shoehorning a break in than it might have been previously, especially for those working from home.

For those working from an office but on screen, it's still important to break the screen time up and ensure you have regular breaks. Don't work through your lunch hour just because you can, it's so easy to do but the only person that doesn't benefit is you.

ASK FOR HELP IF YOU NEED IT

We are all human. If you are struggling with burnout, it may be beneficial to speak to your line manager. They may be able to review your working patterns and amount of time you are on screen.

Consider if you need to take a few days off work while you recover. If you are coping with any additional mental health challenges, don't be afraid to tell someone. Asking for help isn't a sign of weakness, it's a sign you've acknowledged there's a problem and want to do something about it.

OTHER PRACTICAL IDEAS FOR REDUCING SCREEN BURNOUT

- Shorten the length of time you have booked the consultation for, or do it in two shorter sessions. Think about the in-person equivalent and how long you would usually spend during a session, and aim to reduce by 15 minutes at least to allow for additional concentration and the impact of this on the brain in processing, both for the person the session is intended for and the clinician.
- Be focussed. See Section 2 for managing a session, but being organised and prepared could help reduce the length of time actually needed in a session.
- Allow yourself time to step away from your screen. I don't mean walk out half way through a therapy session, but it's OK not to be sat at the desk all day. The camera isn't recording your every move! Just because we are at home, instead of working in a room full of people, doesn't mean

that we are not working hard; in fact, in many instances, it's been reported we are working harder and longer, so we definitely need some time away from the screen.

Don't stop and drop! By this I mean don't stop a video call then go and 'drop' someone an email straight away as you move to tackle your inbox immediately.

We need to use this interlude time to get some fresh air, stretch the legs we forget we have hiding under the desk and hydrate. Make a cup of tea. Do a load of washing, feed the rabbit/cat/dog (all of the them, if you're me). Remember: the longer we sit at screens without a break, the more likely it is that we will succumb to the lure of burnout.

It's Not Wink Murder, So Don't Forget to Blink!
Screens can give you dry eye, and no one wants to deal with the discomfort of that on top of everything else. Over the counter remedies to spray on are available to hydrate itchy, scratchy eyes, but it's important to regularly get your eyes tested. Eye strain can make you feel even more tired and exhausted. Anti-glare coatings might sound like a gimmick but can make a real difference if you are wearing glasses all day, both to the person wearing and those engaging with them. I have recently had my glasses treated for the first time and it's made a big difference to the level of headache I get.

Take Time to Learn the Platform
It may sound obvious, but practice. We wouldn't expect to just know how to do something in any other area of practice, so why would this be any different.

Familiarise yourself with the software's features and functions. What is the process/user experience (UX) for the person joining? Is it different to the joining experience as a clinician?

Have a Few Practice Runs
Whether it's your first time (or even if it's not!), the more you do 'it', the more confident you will feel, and this will translate for the individual and feel more comfortable for them. Even if you've done virtual consultations before, it may be you are

using a different platform for the first time or you're using new online resources and screen sharing, trying different activities or a new session format, practice sending out the link and joining with a colleague or a willing family member. If you are changing screens or moving about the platform and using the features. It's worth it for a more streamlined session and to be able to troubleshoot earlier, too.

Using tech can sometimes go wrong, and in many times, it would be out of your control. It could be a network or Wi-Fi issue. Make sure you know what is in your control and what is not.

- Be careful of your posture. It's easy to slump when you're in a chair at home, but it won't help when you've been sitting like that for seven hours.

Some people I know have a sit/stand desk. It may not be possible where you work, depending on what your set up is, but it can be a good idea to take your laptop with you to different rooms.

HOW'S YOUR HEAD? ENSURING CLINICIAN MENTAL HEALTH AND WELLBEING

It's vitally important to recognise that, although we are the ones delivering the care, we have our own lives happening in the background and virtual care has had an impact on us personally and professionally.

Within our clinical roles taking care of ourselves is essential, whether we are working within a clinic in-person or managing digital clinics or a combination these.

We are increasingly being advised around the power of self-care and using mindfulness as part of this as it is flexible. The 5, 4, 3, 2, 1 approach is a well-documented Grounding Technique (see Figure 49.1). Often used in therapy to manage anxiety, it helps by 'anchoring in the present' to bring our physical and mental selves into synchronicity using the five senses like tethers, anchoring us to the moment. This simple grounding technique can be effectively used when emotions and thoughts become too overwhelming, such as a challenging or emotive therapy session with an individual we are caring for.

The principles are really simple as they don't rely on any complex resources and so can be used whenever and wherever you find yourself needing a wellbeing moment.

Remember, if you have tried self-care but feel you are still in need of more specialist support, contact your GP or local Improving Access to Psychological Therapies (IAPT) service for further advice.

DOI: 10.4324/9781003269724-54

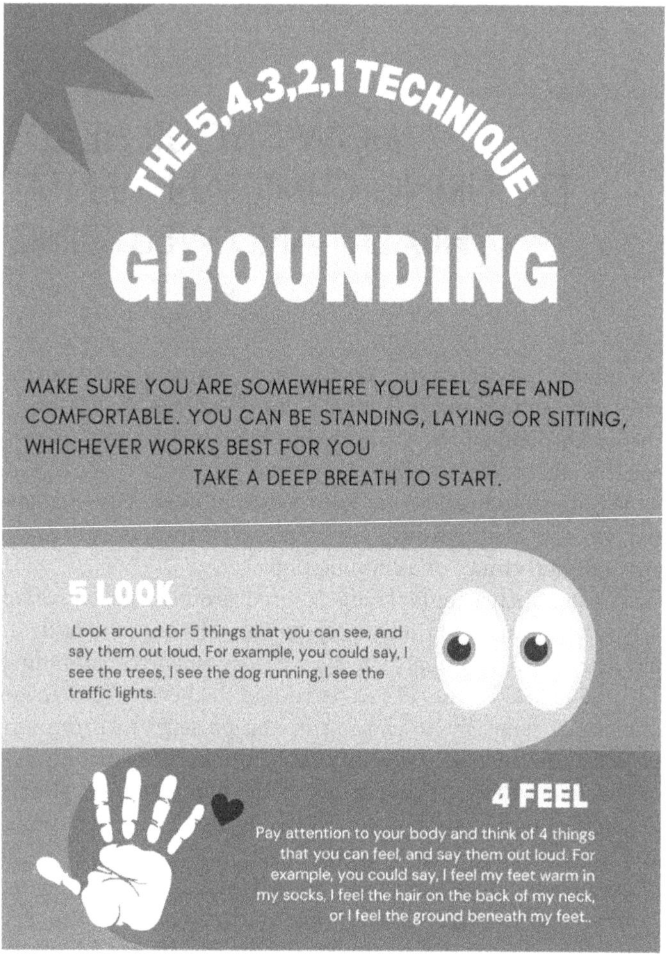

Figure 49.1 5, 4, 3, 2, 1 Grounding Technique

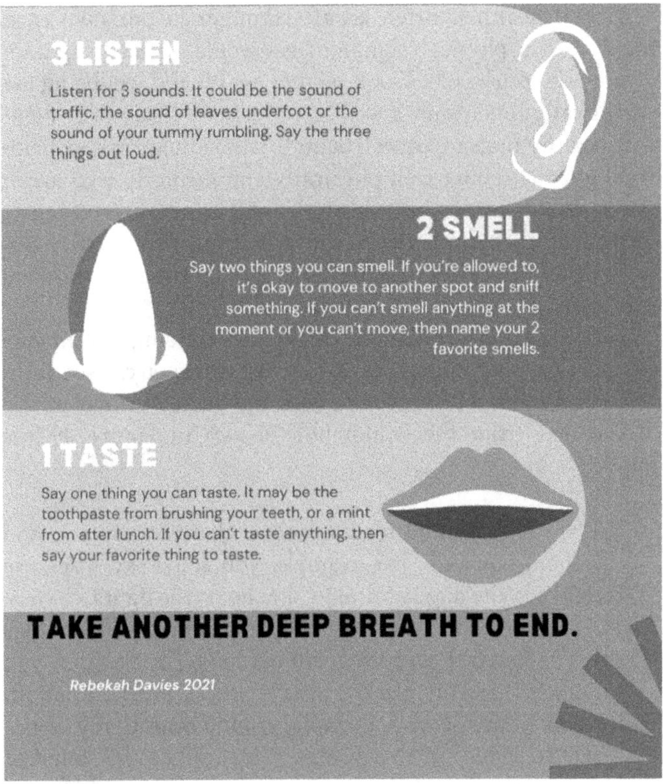

3 LISTEN

Listen for 3 sounds. It could be the sound of traffic, the sound of leaves underfoot or the sound of your tummy rumbling. Say the three things out loud.

2 SMELL

Say two things you can smell. If you're allowed to, it's okay to move to another spot and sniff something. If you can't smell anything at the moment or you can't move, then name your 2 favorite smells.

1 TASTE

Say one thing you can taste. It may be the toothpaste from brushing your teeth, or a mint from after lunch. If you can't taste anything, then say your favorite thing to taste.

TAKE ANOTHER DEEP BREATH TO END.

Rebekah Davies 2021

Figure 49.1 5, 4, 3, 2, 1 Grounding Technique (continued)

Mental health is often an afterthought in our own care, but were it a physical symptom we would be much quicker to attend to our needs. Good mental health and wellbeing are intrinsically linked and 'a well being' is more likely to be mentally healthy than an 'unwell being'! This simple analogy helps highlight that being well physically and mentally well aren't two separate entities but tightly bound together. Working to keep an equilibrium between the two can make positive mental health much easier to achieve but it takes time, practice and awareness of what makes us as individuals tick.

The grounding technique is a really easy and simple technique that can be applied with no resources, just what you can see, hear, touch, feel and smell so it can be used anywhere by anyone.

The text from the infographic shown in Figure 49.1 is detailed below.

5 – LOOK: look around for five things that you can see, and say them out loud. For example, you could say, I see the trees, I see the dog running, I see the traffic lights.
4 – FEEL: pay attention to your body and think of four things that you can feel, and say them out loud. For example, you could say, 'I feel my feet warm in my socks, I feel the hair on the back of my neck, or I feel the ground beneath my feet'.
3 – LISTEN: listen for three sounds. It could be the sound of traffic, the sound of leaves underfoot or the sound of your tummy rumbling. Say the three things out loud.
2 – SMELL: say two things you can smell. If you're allowed to, it's OK to move to another spot and sniff something. If you can't smell anything at the moment or you can't move, then name your two favourite smells.
1 – TASTE: say one thing you can taste. It may be the toothpaste from brushing your teeth, or a mint from after lunch. If you can't taste anything, then say your favourite thing to taste.

Take another deep breath to end.

Some further relaxation activities that may help calm and relax can be found in the resources.

THE REMOTELY POSSIBLE: A VISION FOR A DIGITAL FIRST FUTURE

In 2019 NHS England launched the Long Term Plan, with chapter 5 specific to the digital transformation of the NHS. The vision of this plan was for digital technology to be at the core, to underpin how we provide care so that what we do and how we do it can free up time and create efficiencies and increased interoperability in healthcare. Ultimately this means that we are creating an environment that delivers better outcomes for those we care for by joining different sources of care, ensuring individuals don't have to repeat information over and over again to different clinicians and that we can use digital to do better. This doesn't mean replacing clinicians with robots, digitising every clinical pathway or a patient never setting foot in a clinical setting again. Far from it, it's about making the most appropriate clinical choice based on the individual's needs and choices alongside utilising the best of both in-person and digital interfaces to create the most effective health ecosystem we can possibly deliver.

Essentially do more with less, otherwise known as streamlining! This isn't a euphemism for reducing quality of care, it's a vehicle for enhancing the existing pathways to ensure that an individual receives the most appropriate care for them, in the most timely way, first time, every time. Throughout the duration of the pandemic, waiting lists that were already long were extended even more, particularly in some specialties, meaning services have been further impacted.

Digital tools and pathways provides a potential means to support elective recovery of services and reduce waiting lists

DOI: 10.4324/9781003269724-55

by effective caseload management to filter out some of the individuals waiting that could be offered an alternative route to treatment that is more clinically appropriate and quicker. This is has a two-pronged benefit,

1. Reduction of waiting list/efficient service recovery.
2. Individual can be reviewed to check that what they are waiting for is still relevant, assigned blocks of remote care and/or, they are offered the most appropriate treatment for them as quickly as possible, which may be in-person, remote 1:1 sessions, being prescribed self-monitoring tools or self-managed pathways with the option to initiate an appointment on a Patient Initiated Follow Up pathway (PIFU).

It's important to highlight that, as part of this pathways, if an individual feels they need to see a clinician either sooner than an agreed date or where a date hasn't been agreed, they are able to arrange this using the agreed processes.

This way of managing caseloads using telehealth and hybrid digital services to support someone could make a big difference to the wider recovery of our healthcare systems. Although it has a new name, the approach isn't significantly different in many cases from familiar caseload management strategies SLTs have used historically, it's the tools to manage that may be different.

We have an ageing population, which brings with it more co-morbidities and more need for patients to access healthcare. At the same time, we have critical pressures to address within the system.

Before Covid-19 hit, the Long Term Plan had a vision which was to move 30% of all outpatient appointments to digital care.

Fast forward to 2020, when Covid-19 hit and the digital revolution was thrust upon the market. Most appointments *had* to be virtual. That's not to say it was right for everyone.

The consideration with virtual care is that it absolutely has the potential to help and to have a positive impact, however it has to be done the right way.

Interoperability has always been a challenge for health-care. There are serveal elements to this but one fundamental question is, how do we get multiple systems to integrate with each other to ensure the workflow is simple and easy for both healthcare professionals and patients?

NHS England and NHS Improvement, alongside NHSE/I Transformation Directorate (formerly NHSX) and NHS Digital have been working hard on the Shared Care Record, and INTEROpen are working to ensure suppliers can and will integrate their data, ensuring greater sharing, transparency and accuracy of joined up information. However, even from a technical perspective, with a clear objective and all processes agreed, it just isn't that easy. Transformation on this scale doesn't happen without the relevant resource, capacity and of course a fully formed strategy to map long term objectives to interwoven with all the smaller projects from new digital dic-tation software to remote monitoring and virtual wards to new RPA of administrative processes.

Each healthcare provider has their own unique set up for their Electronic Patient Record (EPR), which makes it harder (but not impossible) for each supplier to integrate. Again it takes time and resources. It is all doable of course, but it isn't as easy as we can sometimes think it will be. It isn't just the flick of a switch or a few buttons and clicks on the keyboard and the whole organisation is suddenly completely streamlined with all its neighbours. This vision is what heathcare systems are striving to achieve long term, to ensure that joined up care is just that, joined up, safe, efficient and interoperable. A digital health eco system where information and data is easily and securely shared and the individual is at the heart of all decision making with the ability to contribute and be part of their own information management. Greenhalgh et al. (2021) highlight in their paper outlining the Planning and Evaluating Remote Consultation Services (PERCS) framework that implementing virtual consulations is part of the wider complexities of digi-tal transformation. Embedding and implementing these ser-vices should be considered within the long terms 'goals' and organisational digital strategies. They allude to considerations around both clinical risk mitigation (Chapter 20) and associated exclusions and the ways in which the framework has potential systemic benefits at multi-levels and for multi-purpose. The acknowledgment that the implications and outcomes are subjective and setting dependent futher highlights that whilst the framework is there to scaffold complex considerations there is no one size fits all approach to this area.

The technology alone is not what makes for transformational change. It is the culmination and application of all of these things together that support the integration of digital pathways. Digital solutions should support our clinical work, provide flexibility, adaptability and inclusivity within our services whilst working towards removing some of the administrative burden we may have acquired additionally associated with the introduction of virtual pathways. Examples such as using Robotic Process Automation (RPA) for sending and analysing feedback forms or to do the validation and 'tech checks' will allow for clinical time to remain as clinical time.

As clinicians, if we can adapt our patient pathways so that the digital solutions complement what we do and aspire to achieve in our services, we could continue to see the success that speech and language therapy and AHP services more broadly, have seen develop at pace over the course of the last few years.

We have begun to acknowledge that we don't need to see every patient for a face-to-face but neither do we need to or should see every patient virtually. It is a hybrid of methods that is most likely to offer the most holistic solution as, no single solution is applicable to all situations .

As Greenhalgh et al. (2021) suggest, the best outcomes in remote consultations should be those which result in the most appriate method of of delivery 'for a particular patient at a particular time'. They also outline that the PERCS framework 'guiding principles will help inform ethical allocation decisions and high-quality remote consulting'.

The quest will ultimately carve out a seamless blend of hybrid healthcare delivery that utilises both in-person, virtual and remote pathways synchronously and asynchronously.

Digital will enable more efficient use of time and clinical prioritisations allowing for in-person encounters that are supported and acknowledged by framworks such as those outlined in specific relation to virtual delivery, whilst driven by the broader digital objectives of the NHS Long Term Plan and associated national agendas for digital transformation.

The digital journey of speech and language is just at the precipice, there is much to learn and achieve and it is part of something so much bigger and more complex but, there are goals, aspirations, and structure underpinning the work required. The NHS Long Term Plan with the addition of the new Patient Safety and Digital Clinical Safety Strategies and DTAC with the introduction of remote consultation specific frameworks including the PERCS are resources to support, scaffold and steer the understanding, implementation, adoption and sustainability of new technologies, processes and pathways.

A hybrid methodology of delivery not only creates the conditions for delivering care at the right time by the right method but also encourages increased self-direction by individuals who may be more engaged, autonomous and have accountability for their own healthcare when they are provided with the tools to do so. Individuals are equipped with the tools and options for how, when, who and where they engage, offering increased flexibility around employment, families and busy lives. The focus rather than managing illness will be encouraging wellness.There are several initiatives that will use digital tools as enablers to drive them including the new NHS England and NHS Improvement My Planned Care service launched in February 2022 which will also align with the NHS app. All of these together, impact longer term as, for some clinicians, care will take a less directive approach as 'People will be helped to stay well, to recognise important symptoms early, and to manage their own health, guided by digital tools' (NHS Long Term Plan, chapter 5 – 5.8). This may be the case to some extent for speech and language therapy, that individuals will increasingly make use of digital tools to support and manage their needs but clinicians will also adapt to the changes in demands and make the most efficient use of digital pathways flexing and changing with the landscape to deliver interventions that meet the needs of the individuals.

There are factors which remain unchanged however, wherever and whenever we deliver therapy. The core of what it means to be a speech and language therapist is to not only have a specialist clinical knowledge, expertise and insight unique to our discipline but to have a compassion and passion that is immeasurable and quite literally enables us to 'give voice' to those who need us most. These will always be required in order that we are able to holistically manage the needs of individuals and support them at home, work or in education.

CAREER PROGRESSION

On a very practical level, healthcare will continue to change, to adapt, flex and blend the best of all approaches. This is simply a fact. Change happens. National agencies are paving the way through the ongoing revision of existing frameworks and the development of new strategy and policy to guide and shape progress. There are many places to access more information and progress your knowledge about digital health or even consider pursing as a career pathway. There is information specific to both speech and language therapy and the wider digital agenda including RCSLT who have an informatics department and manage a regular telehealth e-bulletin, whilst Health Education England and their digital readiness programme is much broader. Much of the information is open access, but to apply for their training and development programmes you must be directly employed by the NHS. Their programmes include the Topol Digital Health Fellowship and NHS Digital Academy with Imperial College London. There are also localised training and development courses, including the Digital Health London Pioneer programme. If you are looking for support and inspiration from like minded clinicians, the Shuri Network (see also Chapter 3) is a supportive award winning network for BAME women in health tech but anyone who is interested in their community can join as an ally and the growing, innovative and inspirational community is always open. Search Shuri Network or @NetworkShuri on Twitter for more information.

If it is more of an academic route that interests you and you might consider research around an aspect of digital health and its impact, then the National Institute for Health Research (NIHR) is a useful source of information as they host several programmes, including a foundation stage programme into academic study. Many of these links can be found in the resources or by searching the organisation name in your preferred browser.

DATA REALLY DOES SAVE LIVES

Data is a significant part of transformation and of the future of digital practice. It informs improvements and supports recommendations and business cases. It can also save lives. It is the evidence base of healthcare and where there is a pathway, process or person there is data to be collated. From feed back forms and radiotherapy outcomes and discharge to own home vs discharge to care, to number of patients admitted at weekends for swallow assessments, the data we collate can help us improve, adapt and even prevent the same or similar occurrences happening again by understanding the data. Risk mitigation is central to digital work and it is the underlying data that is the driver, preventer, enabler and saviour.

Granular level data not only serves to build an intricate jigsaw of interlinked information but, it inform the safety and strategy of digital clinical assurance in the deployment of technology across and within specialities. Together we can begin to shape this work, inform the future of care whilst ensuring the integrity and security of information that we share.

As we continue to move towards a digitally enabled future within health it is becoming recognised that a clinically led but person-centred and directed approach is needed to maximise accessibility, efficacy and drive forward innovation. Care that is directed by and with the needs of the patient, enhanced and enabled by digital tools to optimise the potential of integrated and interoperable care will result in healthcare that is not only safe but effective and efficient.

The vision for the future of healthcare remains much the same as it is now in that the person being cared for should be at the heart of care and this hasn't changed, but we have learned it is the fundamentals enabling this vision of care that has. From video consultations and dedicated software that supports them, to tens of thousands of heathcare apps, online resources and wearable devices, digital tools are just one enabler.

We as digital clinicians and practitioners are also enablers. Skilled in supporting individuals and groups to engage using digital means, communicate and manage administrative tasks with enhanced digital elements to integrate and streamline delivery.

We have already learned that clinical care is more flexible than anyone believed it could possibly be even just a short time ago, imagine then the future of care where individuals are provided more autonomy and input about the way in which their care is delivered. This is not only a possibility in the future but the vision for the future (The NHS Long Term Plan, 2019), and although we are still navigating and learning, we are a strong, creative and innovative community discovering that speech and language therapy in its many varied forms is above all most definitely, remotely possible!

INDEX

For Product Safety Concerns and Information please contact our EU
representative GPSR@taylorandfrancis.com
Taylor & Francis Verlag GmbH, Kaufingerstraße 24, 80331 München, Germany